MW01231819

Lose Weight

with

LCHF

The

Low-Carb-High-Fat

"Diet"

Blue Elephant Publishing
Copyright © 2012 by Eric Ahlswede
All rights reserved

Lose Weight with LCHF:

The Low-Carb-High-Fat "Diet"

(Rated PG Edition)

By Eric Ahlswede

Blue Elephant Publishing
Box 94, 414/20 Moo. 12
Nongprue, Banglamung
Chonburi, Thailand
20150

Blue Elephant Publishing
6457 North Star Rd.
Ferndale, WA
United States
98248-8613

loseweightwithlchf.com
blueelephantpublishing.com

All rights reserved. This book is sold subject to the condition that it shall not, by way of trade or otherwise, be lent, resold, hired out or otherwise circulated, in any form of binding or cover, without the author's prior written consent. No part of this book may be reproduced by any process, nor may the book be transmitted or otherwise copied for public or private use without the written permission of the author. Although the author has made every reasonable attempt to achieve complete accuracy of the content in this book, the author assumes no responsibility for errors or omissions. Any trademarks, service marks, product names or named features are assumed to be the property of their respective owners, and are used only for reference. There is no implied endorsement of these terms.

Copyright © 2012 by Eric Ahlswede

ISBNs:

978-1-62506-000-6

978-1-62506-001-3

978-1-62506-002-0

978-1-62506-003-7

978-1-62506-004-4

978-1-62506-005-1

978-1-62506-006-8

978-1-62506-007-5

978-1-62506-008-2

978-1-62506-009-9

First Printing 2012

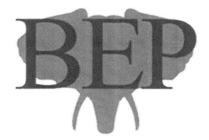

Table of Contents

FOREWORD

By: John Kendall

Eric Ahlswede, the author of this book, and I first became friends in Costa Rica in 1997. We'd met at a pub called *The Beatle Bar* where I ran a karaoke show. Eric sang well enough and became a regular customer. We were soon close friends, singing classic rock songs and playing golf together.

Eric now lives in Thailand and truly enjoys living there. It pleases me to say that I was the one that introduced him to that country. Though I live in Costa Rica, I visit Thailand several times a year.

This year, 2012, I visited Thailand again and looked Eric up. We agreed to have breakfast together at a local expat restaurant called *Rich Man Poor Man*. He looked me over and said that while I looked well enough, he noticed I'd put on a bit of weight. I admitted that my weight had increased to 224 pounds. I'm 6 feet 2 inches tall, and 224 pounds is too much. I like to be about 200 pounds. In the past when my weight climbed, I'd go on what I call a "diet" and begin to exercise more. It usually took a couple of months of hard work and a little food deprivation to do so, but I always lost the weight. Last year my attempt at weight loss wasn't so successful. I'm 62 years old now and it seems that age had caught up with me. I couldn't drop weight like I had in the past.

Over breakfast, Eric seemed eager to share something with me. He told me that he'd been researching health and weight loss. He told me his research would apply to me. He spoke of a low-carb-high-fat diet called LCHF. I listened, as I've always known him to be a sincere, intelligent and energetic person.

What he told me was absolutely contrary to what I knew about health and weight loss. I thought a bowl of granola, toast without butter, orange juice and coffee with a little sugar was a good start to the day. Maybe eggs at times, but certainly no bacon.

Eric told me I had it all wrong. He told me to eat saturated fats. He said I could eat anytime I wanted, as long as I didn't eat carbohydrates. Eric was pretty convincing. I decided to give LCHF a try. Plus, what did I have to lose. No pun intended.

Before I got on LCHF, I weighed 224 pounds. Five weeks later, using LCHF, I weighed 209 pounds. Another four weeks later on LCHF and I'm down to 200 pounds. That's 24 pounds in 9 weeks.

LCHF works! I feel good, and I've received some very nice compliments on my new physique. I'm very grateful to Eric.

Back in Costa Rica, I wasn't on LCHF. I'd never heard of it. I used the gym in Costa Rica, but struggled with weight loss. Here in Thailand, I'm on LCHF, but I don't go to the gym. Weight loss on LCHF is a breeze. I must admit that I walked various golf courses 20 times during my 9 weeks of LCHF, but no gym time.

So, to recap, I'm exercising less, drinking alcohol more (hey, I'm on vacation) and I'm losing weight with LCHF. I'm eating steaks, pork chops, eggs and bacon. I try to eat green vegetables, but I no longer eat carbohydrates. At Eric's suggestion, I switched to low-carb beer. I'm never hungry and I never feel deprived. LCHF works and I plan to stick with it. I hope you read his book. LCHF changed my life. It can change yours.

Sincerely,

John Kendall
Escazu, Costa Rica

DISCLAIMER

Warning

I designed this book to provide you with information on a better way of eating. I sold the book to you with the understanding that I'm not engaged in rendering medical, legal, or any professional services. If you require those services, get a professional.

I'm here to educate and entertain. I'm here to give you explanations and anecdotes about a way of eating that changed my life. Learn what you can from these explanations and anecdotes. Make an *informed* decision on what foods you're going to put in your body. It's your choice.

Rated PG Edition

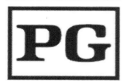

I'd never had any interest in *reading* self-help books. Most seemed boring. When I decided to write this book, I thought I'd spice things up a bit by including some *risqué* tales of living abroad. I thought I'd give the book some *personality*.

I've lived a very active life. Many of the explanations and anecdotes in this edition, *Lose Weight with LCHF: The Low-Carb-High-Fat "Diet" (Rated PG Edition),* could be considered offensive to some people as they include mild profanity. As I came closer to finishing this book, it dawned on me that my profanity may be offensive to a large demographic.

I thought about it for a while, then created a less profane edition, a *Rated*-G edition. If you find *risqué* tales and mild profanity offensive, you might try the *Lose Weight with LCHF: The Low-Carb-High-Fat "Diet" (Rated G Edition).*

WEBSITE

Website

Most websites I visit during my day are poorly designed, contain too much content and are difficult to navigate. I wanted the website for this book to be different. I wanted the website for this book to be clean and easy to use. I wrote and designed **loseweightwithlchf.com** using Apple's iWeb. I then contracted with Tony Ham of tonyhamCREATIVE[1] to polish it up and make it functional for use on SquareSpace[2], the host. Tony did an amazing job. He took my rough draft and created something quite special.

Please visit **loseweightwithlchf.com**. Contact me. I'd like to hear your thoughts and your experiences. If LCHF improved your life, help me spread the word. Tell your friends and family to visit **loseweightwithlchf.com** and buy the book.

---

1   www.tonyhamcreative.com
2   www.squarespace.com

6

PREFACE

Finding LCHF

In 2010 I traveled from my home in Thailand to Costa Rica to visit old friends and look after investments. One day, I was walking on the beaches of Esterillos where a friend snapped my photo. When I saw the photo, I was appalled. Who was that fat guy? My physique truly surprised me. I knew I was getting bigger, buying *fat-pants* for every trip to the U.S., I just didn't know how big.

The week after that, I was visiting a friend in Aurora, CO. We had a lot of fun the first few days, but one night we just wanted to relax. My friend had a Netflix account, so I previewed the films, focusing on documentaries. I choose one film, entitled *Fat Head,* by Tom Naughton.

Fat Head began as a rebuttal to another documentary, *Super Size Me,* by Morgan Spurlock. However, *Fat Head* finished with explanations detailing the harm caused by carbohydrates and the benefits provided by saturated fats. This latter part of *Fat Head* appealed to my logic. I decided to make a change. I *reduced* my intake of carbohydrates and I *increased* my intake of saturated fats.

I ate beef, pork, chicken and green vegetables. I ate 4 or 5 eggs every day. I cooked with bacon grease, butter and olive oil. *Unsweetened* whipping cream was soon my favorite additive.

I no longer ate foods containing high amounts of carbohydrates. I no longer ate bread, pasta, rice, breakfast cereals, soft drinks, fruit juices or desserts. Whenever I was hungry, I satisfied my hunger with foods containing saturated fats. Pork chops, steaks, chicken wings, bacon, eggs and cheese.

Can you guess what happened? The answers might surprise you. I lost 30 pounds. I slept better. I had more energy. My blood pressure dropped. My blood chemistry improved. This damn thing worked!

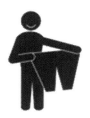

The results were so immediate and surprising, I started to really dig into this thing. I researched, deeper and deeper. I read books, online articles, blogs, threads and forums.

I was driving my friends crazy with conversations and emails extolling this style of eating. Several friends suggested I stop writing emails and begin writing a book. This book is the result of my continuing research and the wishes of my friends. A warning though, this book is not your typical diet book.

Dedication

This book is dedicated to Tom Naughton. His movie, *Fat Head*, helped me find LCHF. Thanks Tom.

Acknowledgements

Dr. Annika Dahlqvist, Njurunda, Sweden. Thank you Dr. Dahlqvist for showing us the way.

Dr. Andreas Eenfeldt, Karlstad, Sweden. Thank you Dr. Eenfeldt for your kind, informative responses to my inquiries.

Cindy Kausek, Gonzales, LA, USA. Thanks for your amazing copyediting and helping find my way out of run-on-sentences and to recognize split infinitives.

Kay Faulkner, Ferndale, WA, USA. Thanks for your meticulous proofreading and being "Mom #2."

Ann Ahlswede, Pleasanton, CA, USA. Thanks, "Lil' Sis," for your thoughts, hopes and organization of my stick-figures and icons.

Julia Mallonee, Aurora, CO, USA. Thanks for allowing me to put a chapter in my book about the friend we both lost.

Lisa & Mike Smith, Issaquah, WA, USA. Thanks for your ever present support and your responses to my many inquiries on the weight you both lost.

"Wild Bill" Wichrowski, Kodiak, AK, USA. Thanks, pardner, for letting me include you.

"Big Dick Steve" Poznanski, Pattaya, Thailand. Thanks, wild man, for letting me use your photos and stories.

"Karaoke John" Kendall, Escazu, Costa Rica. Thanks, you big lug, for letting me use your photos and data on weight loss.

"Arturo" O'Connor, Jomtien, Thailand. Thanks, Art. Your continued weight loss impresses us all.

Steve Martini, Bellingham, WA, USA. Thanks for sharing lunch with me and giving me your input on how the book industry works.

John Lafond Wright, Pattaya, Thailand. Thanks for the great photos.

Craig Matthews, Pattaya, Thailand. Thanks, partner, for your enthusiasm and help with the book title.

Tim Manley, Na Jomtien, Thailand. Thanks for your thoughtful input and your free beer.

Finally, a special thanks to my friend who wishes to remain unnamed. Thanks for poking and prodding me into writing down my thoughts and research.

I'd also like to thank those folks I've never met in person, but whose help was invaluable.

Tengku Rahmaddansyah, Medan, Sumatera, Indonesia. Thank you "T." for the technical assistance with logos and icons.

Megan McCullough, Steger, IL, USA. Thank you for your help and research in preparing this book for publication.

Tony Ham, tonyhamCREATIVE[3]. Thank you for creating an amazing website.

Joel Friedlander, The Book Designer[4]. Thank you for providing me with an amazing tool, *10 Things You Need to Know About Self-Publishing.*

Dan Poynter, ParaPublishing[5]. Thank you for providing me with your book on self-publishing, *Self-Publishing Manual: How to Write, Print and Sell Your Own Book.*

The folks at BookCoverPro[6]. Thank you for creating an amazing application.

---

3 www.tonyhamcreative.com
4 www.thebookdesigner.com
5 www.parapublishing.com
6 www.bookcoverpro.com

The folks at Shutterstock[7]. Thank you for providing me with hundreds of photos, icons and graphics.

The folks at Hover[8]. Thank you for providing me with a simple, elegant domain management site.

7   www.shutterstock.com

8   www.hover.com

ABOUT THE AUTHOR

My "Qualifications"

I'm a complete composite of my parents. I gained mathematical, mechanical and logic skills from my father. I gained organizational, commonsense and love-of-life skills from my mother.

I live life hard, loving, laughing and drinking more than most. I rarely worry, almost never lose my temper and truly enjoy the company of others. I'm a very bright, very outgoing, open-minded *man-child* with *no* medical training. I can problem-solve. I'm great with numbers. I know how to research and I can usually see through *bullshit*.

Does any of this *qualify* me to author a book about weight loss and improved health? *Should you read what I have to say?* Maybe not, but I promise to light up your logic and even entertain you.

My Earlier Years

I'm an American male of Teutonic bloodline, born and raised in Racine, Wisconsin. I spent the first 6 years of my adulthood as an auxiliary-equipment engineer in the U.S. Navy. I was GI-Bill educated in Washington State and have a career background in international tax law and finance.

My Recent Years

I was lucky enough to semi-retire at the age of 44. I began my retirement in 2000, moving to Costa Rica and living there for the next five years.

Following an exploratory golf trip to East Asia, I moved to Thailand in 2005 and have lived here since. Thailand is amazing. Thailand is called *The Land of Smiles*. The people of Thailand are kind, generous and thoughtful. I hope to live here for the rest of my life. I wrote this book in Thailand.

My Weight Gain

In high school I was one of those tall, gangly guys, 6'2" and 165 pounds. Post high school, I enlisted in the U.S. Navy. I finished boot-camp at 185 pounds.

Every year following, I would add a pound or two, primarily around my middle. Every year, my weight and cholesterol got higher. Every year, my libido and energy got lower. Every year, my body experienced changes.

These changes didn't really bother me. I just assumed these changes were the consequences of getting older. I now know differently. These changes were the consequences of a lifetime of eating carbohydrates.

I no longer eat many carbohydrates. I now eat saturated fats. This simple change in diet has dramatically improved my life. I'm thinner and healthier. I'm thinking more clearly and getting more done. I have higher energy and libido. I'm happier. I'm young again.

Writing this book

I'd always been told that I write well. However, when I began writing this book, my wording was terrible, my sentence structure was awful. I had trouble presenting ideas in a logical and palatable form. My writing skills had deteriorated.

I think I know the cause. My writing skills had deteriorated because I live in Thailand. When speaking to Thais who have limited knowledge of English, I often switch to a *pidgin-style* of communicating. It's not unusual for me to say, "What you do? Where you go? I go bar now." Hopefully you'll give me a pass if I stumble on a phrase or two.

It should also be noted that I wrote this book using general-public vernacular. I wanted the LCHF explanations and anecdotes to be clear and easily understood by all. There are many fine books on low-carbohydrate eating that were written in a more formal style, an example being Gary Taubes[9], *Why We Get Fat*[10]. I simply

---

9   garytaubes.com

10 garytaubes.com/works/books/why-we-get-fat/

wished to write a book that was informative, yet lyrical and entertaining.

I used Post-it notes to organize the chapters of this book. A Thai friend of mine saw my wall of Post-it notes and asked what they were for. I explained that I was writing a book about eating the right foods and *not* eating the wrong foods. With much difficulty, I asked her to guess how many words my book contained. Her response was, "One million." She was a little off, the book finished up around 40,000 words. I've tried to make this book concise, educational and entertaining.

"I would have written a shorter letter, but I did not have the time."

- Blaise Pascal, Lettres Provinciales, Letter XVI

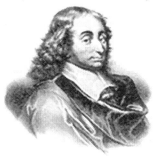

Blaise Pascal (1623-1662)

INTRODUCTION

LCHF

My *father's father* was 55 years old when he died of heart disease. In a morbid coincidence my *father* was 55 years old when he died of heart disease. I suspect that the culprits in both deaths were refined carbohydrates. I had no wish to die when I became 55, so I choose LCHF.

Q.: What do ranchers feed their cattle to prepare them for market?

A.: Cattle are fed grain containing carbohydrates a few months before slaughter to dramatically increase the animals' weight and intramuscular fat.

Q.: What does a mother feed her hungry baby?

A.: A hungry baby is fed milk containing saturated fat to alleviate the baby's hunger and ensure growth and development of the baby's body and mind.

LCHF stands for Low-Carbohydrate-High-Fat. LCHF is easy. You simply replace the carbohydrates in your diet with saturated fats. You eat whenever you're hungry. You stop eating when you're not. There's no need for exercise or starvation.

The title of this book is *Lose Weight with LCHF: The Low-Carb-High-Fat "Diet."* With LCHF, you may eat as much as you like, any time you like. LCHF is *not* a diet. LCHF is a way of eating. This is why the word "Diet" is in quotation marks in the book's subtitle.

The goal of this book is to educate you on a different way of eating, the LCHF way of eating. In *Lose Weight with LCHF: The Low-Carb-High-Fat "Diet,"* you'll learn solutions toward lower weight, better health, higher energy and clearer thinking.

Here's what you'll discover in *Lose Weight with LCHF: The Low-Carb-High-Fat "Diet"*

- Why LCHF helps you lose weight and keep it off
- Which foods to eat and which foods to avoid
- Which health *problems* are caused by eating carbohydrates
- Which health *benefits* are gained by eating saturated fats

15

LCHF Origins

LCHF stands for Low-Carbohydrate-High-Fat. I wanted to present the origins of LCHF in this book, so I made a Wikipedia search of "LCHF." My search was rewarded with the following: *"The LHCf ("Large Hadron Collider forward") is a special-purpose Large hadron Collider experiment for astroparticle (cosmic ray) physics, and one of seven detectors in the LHC accelerator at CERN."* The LCHF I'll be discussing does not require a cosmic ray.

Low-carbohydrate diets have been around for some time. However, low-carbohydrate-**high-fat** diets are fairly new. LCHF, low-carbohydrate-high-fat, seems to have originated in Sweden by Dr. Annika Dahlqvist. The doctor developed a theory that her obese and diabetic patients shouldn't *ignore* their energy needs by eating limited amounts of low-fat carbohydrates. The doctor thought her patients should *acknowledge* their energy needs by eating foods their bodies were designed to process. Saturated fats.

It worked. Her obese patients eating saturated fats in place of low-fat carbohydrates quickly reduced weight. Her diabetic patients eating saturated fats in place of low-fat carbohydrates quickly reduced blood sugar and had less need for insulin.

Maybe this theory of acknowledging energy needs with saturated fats would apply to *all* patients. Maybe this theory would apply to *everyone.*

Of course you know what happened when it became public knowledge that a physician was prescribing saturated fats as a path towards better health. The medical community went nuts. They attacked her and tried to get her medical license yanked. Those knuckleheads didn't care that the doctor's patients were becoming slimmer and healthier. They stuck to their mantra, "Fat is bad!"

She fought back and a public debate ensued, a debate that was lengthy and heated. The Swedish government looked into it. They conducted a detailed investigation and found in Dr. Dahlqvist favor. She was first vilified and then later praised. The Swedish public embraced the doctor's theory. The LCHF movement was born.

LCHF FAQs

Here are a few questions I'm most often asked.

Is There an LCHF Action-Plan?

Everything I've read about writing a self-help book says that the book should always begin with an *action-plan*. OK, here's the *action-plan* for LCHF: Replace the carbohydrates in your diet with saturated fats. Eat whenever you're hungry. Stop eating when you're not.

What Should I Eat?

Whether you exercise or not, your body needs energy to function. There are two food groups that supply energy, carbohydrates and fat. You've got to satisfy your energy needs with *one or both* of these food groups or you'll starve. You *should* eat saturated fats and green vegetables. You *shouldn't* eat carbohydrates.

Who Will Benefit From LCHF?

LCHF is for everyone, providing benefits to all. If you're overweight, LCHF will help you lose weight. If you have high blood sugar, LCHF will help you lower it. If your cholesterol is bad, LCHF will help you raise your *good-cholesterol* and lower your *bad-cholesterol*. If you're simply tired, LCHF will help you raise your energy level.

LCHF will benefit the overweight and the thin. LCHF will benefit both men and women. LCHF will benefit the young, the middle-aged and the old. You gotta fit into one of these categories.

Is LCHF Difficult?

Now the best part. LCHF is easy. You don't have to starve and you don't have to exercise. With LCHF you'll lose weight and improve your health just by eating the right foods and *not* eating the wrong foods. It worked for me. It worked for my friends.

LCHF IN BRIEF

"Saturated fats make you healthy.
Carbohydrates make you fat."

LCHF & Weight

When you eat LCHF, you eat less because the energy in the food you eat will be *used*. Conversely, when you eat carbohydrates, you eat more because much of the energy in the food you eat will be *stored*. Here's a breakdown.

Weight Gain

- Carbohydrates raise blood sugar
- Raised blood sugar causes insulin production
- Insulin causes energy to be *stored*
- Insulin doesn't allow stored energy to be released
- Stored energy that can't be released means weight gain
- Saturated fats don't cause insulin production
- Saturated fats cause energy to be *used*

LCHF will make your body function as it's been designed to function. You won't *store* energy, you'll *use* energy. Because you're eating foods that you've been designed to eat, your body will become efficient. You won't feel the need to eat as often.

LCHF & Health

You may ask, "What about my health?" Saturated fats improve your health. Carbohydrates harm your health. Here are the breakdowns.

Heart Disease

- Carbohydrates cause inflammation
- Inflammation causes cholesterol production
- Carbohydrates cause cholesterol production of the wrong pattern
- The wrong pattern of cholesterol becomes oxidized
- Oxidized cholesterol means heart disease

- Saturated fats don't cause cholesterol production of the wrong pattern of cholesterol
- Saturated fats don't cause oxidized cholesterol that becomes heart disease

Diabetes
- Carbohydrates cause raised blood sugar
- Raised blood sugar causes insulin production
- Repeated insulin production causes unresponsive cells
- Unresponsive cells can't lower blood sugar
- Blood sugar that can't be lowered means diabetes
- Saturated fats don't cause insulin production
- Saturated fats don't cause diabetes

Blood Fats
- Carbohydrates cause lower HDL (good) cholesterol
- Carbohydrates cause higher LDL (bad) cholesterol
- Carbohydrates cause unhealthy cholesterol profiles
- Saturated fats cause higher HDL (good) cholesterol
- Saturated fats cause lower LDL (bad) cholesterol
- Saturated fats cause healthy cholesterol profiles

You've got to satisfy your energy needs or you'll remain hungry. LCHF will satisfy your energy needs with foods that *don't* cause heart disease or diabetes. LCHF will satisfy your energy needs with foods that raise your *good-cholesterol* and lower your *bad-cholesterol*.

LCHF & Cholesterol

The most common response I get when proposing a diet rich in saturated fats and low in carbohydrates is a hysterical, "But what about my cholesterol?!" So, let's get this important question out of the way and alleviate any fears you may have. Here are two statements of fact.

1. Eating saturated fats raises your HDL (*good-cholesterol*) and lowers your LDL (*bad-cholesterol*).

2. Eating carbohydrates raises your LDL (*bad-cholesterol)* and lowers your HDL (*good-cholesterol).*

I eat 4 or 5 eggs every day. I eat a lot of meat, butter and green vegetables. I use heavy, *unsweetened* whipping cream in many dishes and drinks. I love the stuff and go through a pint or so a week. I *don't* eat carbohydrates. My HDL (High-Density Lipoprotein), also known as the *good-cholesterol,* is usually about 100. What's yours?

Embrace the LCHF way of eating with no worries. LCHF improves your health and the chemistry of your blood. Don't believe arguments to the contrary. Everything we've been taught about cholesterol is dead wrong. Foods high in saturated fat *do not* raise your *bad-cholesterol.* Foods high in saturated fat *do* raise your *good-cholesterol.*

ผลการตรวจทางเคมีคลินิก (Blood Chemistry)			Normal range	Comment
Sugar (Glucose)	90	(mg%)	70 - 110	
BUN (Kidney Function Test)	11	(mg%)	5-25	
Creatinine (Kidney Function Test)	0.9	(mg%)	0.5 - 1.5	
Uric acid (For Gout Disease)	4.8	(mg%)	2.0 - 7.5	
Cholesterol (Lipid)	253	(mg%)	150 - 200	[H]
Triglyceride (Lipid)	98	(mg%)	30 - 170	
HDL-C (Lipid)	102	(mg%)	>35	
LDL-C (Lipid)	131	(mg%)	<150	
SGOT (AST) (Liver Function Test)	22	(IU/L)	<40	
SGPT (ALT) (Liver Function Test)	14	(IU/L)	<40	
Alk.phos (Liver Function Test)	43	(IU/L)	25 - 90	
Remark : Found Total Cholesterol higher than normal range				

My recent blood test results.

Did you notice that my Total Cholesterol of 253 was tagged as [H], high. The software used to tag test results ignored the fact that my HDL of 102 pushed the Total Cholesterol above the "Normal Range." If my HDL was 35, a figure typical for a person eating carbohydrates, my Total Cholesterol would have been 166, well within the "Normal Range."

My *good-cholesterol* is 300% of that of a person eating carbohydrates, yet the software was programmed to tag *me* as the one with the health risk. The medical community, government, family, friends, films and television continuously reinforce our misconceptions.

"Excuse me, you guys down here hear about the ongoing cholesterol problem in the country?"

- Vinny Gambini in My Cousin Vinny (1992), as played by Joe Pesci

You *shouldn't* be afraid of producing *either* LDL or HDL cholesterol. Your body fights inflammation with LDL and removes the exhausted cholesterol with HDL.

You *should* be afraid of cholesterol that *becomes* oxidized. Oxidized cholesterol is the plaque that narrows your arteries. Carbohydrates cause cholesterol to become oxidized. Saturated fats don't.

If you'd like to learn specifics about cholesterol before beginning LCHF, refer to the chapter entitled Advanced Discussion of Cholesterol.

Make Informed Decisions

Make informed decisions about what you put into your body. Be prepared to challenge what you read and what you hear as you go throughout your day. There's a lot of misinformation out there. Use tools like Google, Wikipedia and Snopes to gather information and challenge what you hear and see. Try to obtain both or all sides of a story. Digest the information and only then come to an *informed* decision.

Completely ignore *scare-emails*. I've researched dozens of these malicious writings and they're never true. Tell your friends to stop forwarding that crap to you. I had to block one friend's email, as he was hitting that Forward button too often.

It's difficult to be objective with information that's *contrary* to your existing beliefs. When it comes to your health, keep an open mind. Don't stick to a set of beliefs just because you've held those beliefs for years. Don't always believe dogma, it's often wrong. An example might be the idea that foods high in cholesterol are bad for you. That's dead wrong.

If you find a term you don't understand, look it up. This is easily accomplished by typing "define [term you want to look up]" in your Google search window. If you want a more detailed explanation, try Wikipedia. One of the great things about Wikipedia is that the information is fairly current, often reviewed and includes links to sources.

I have hundreds of hours of research in this book. I've read medical journals, medical articles, online articles, blogs and forums. Sources led to other sources. Links led to other links. The chain of research grew and grew. I tried to be thoroughly informed as I wrote this book.

Even though this book is a summary of this research, you still might like to do a bit of research on your own. *Challenge what I've written.* This will increase your understanding of LCHF.

IMPLEMENTING LCHF

"LCHF is easy.
You stop eating carbohydrates and start eating saturated fats."

LCHF Basics

LCHF stands for Low-Carbohydrate-High-Fat. It is a way of eating and not a *diet* in the traditional sense. Traditional *diets* starve your body into weight loss. They're dangerous and never, ever produce *permanent* weight loss. Not without chronic hunger.

LCHF is a way of eating, a way that you should incorporate into your life each and every day. Some folks even refer to LCHF as a *life-style.*

LCHF is simple. You stop eating refined carbohydrates and start eating saturated fats.

- **Eat:** Meat, fish, poultry, eggs and green vegetables.
- **Use:** Olive oil, butter and cream. Even bacon grease and artificial sweeteners are OK.
- **Don't Eat:** Bread, pasta, rice, breakfast cereals, oatmeal, soft drinks, fruit juices or desserts. Eat nothing containing sugar or foods that your body converts to sugar.
- **Don't Use:** Oils containing trans-fats.
- **Eat in Moderation:** Fruits, nuts and alcohol.

Eat any time you're hungry. Stop eating when you're not. Your fat cells will become *retrained* and your weight will drop. Your body will adjust to the change and your health will improve. It's really that simple.

Eating LCHF style *doesn't* mean you're allowed to consume huge amounts of saturated fats. These foods are too rich in calories. Eating LCHF *does* mean that you should replace carbohydrates with *enough* saturated fats to alleviate your hunger.

You'll be surprised at how controlled your appetite will become. You won't be hungry all the time. You'll have a lot more energy. Your body will become efficient.

"The Proof is in the Pudding." This proverb is a shortened version of the original: "The proof of the pudding is in the eating." The proverb dates back to 1615. It means that you can only judge the value of something by *utilizing* that something. You may believe what you've read and researched, but to really judge the value of LCHF, you've got to utilize LCHF. Give it a try.

Beginning LCHF

Before you begin LCHF, you'll want to know where you've started. You'll want to know your *initial* weight, body fat percentage, blood chemistry and level of well being. If you don't know where you've started, how can you know how far you've come?

(1) Determine weight and body fat percentage. I suggest you buy one of those advanced bathroom scales that have four contact plates for your feet. Buying a scale of this type isn't necessary, but they're inexpensive at around $40. I didn't buy one of these scales until six months into LCHF and now wish I'd purchased one much earlier.

(2) Determine blood chemistry. I suggest you get a blood test showing lipid profiles. You want to know your *initial* Total Cholesterol, HDL, LDL and Triglycerides.

(3) Determine your level of well being. I suggest you make specific notes. You should write down your state of mind, your energy level and your physical comfort or discomfort. Be honest with yourself. How do you *really* feel?

If you're concerned that eating LCHF style is going to adversely affect your health, I suggest you get a thorough checkup before you begin. Explain to your doctor what you're going to do. Tell your doctor that you plan on replacing the carbohydrates in your diet with saturated fats. Ask your doctor if there are any grave dangers *specific to you* in trying this style of eating for 60 days.

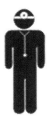

Note to Diabetics: Diabetics have to be a little careful when beginning LCHF. Eating LCHF means your body will no longer produce much insulin. Any blood sugar lowering medication

26

you're still taking could result in blood sugar that's too low. Diabetics beginning LCHF should continuously monitor their blood sugar.

Monitor your Progress

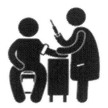

Try to obtain your weight and body fat percentage every few *days* or so. Try to obtain your blood chemistry every few *months* or so. Compare these figures to those you obtained when you began LCHF. If the results aren't as you wish, scale down on the number of carbohydrates you're eating.

When I began LCHF, I didn't really have much to go on. I had a few old blood tests, an old bathroom scale and a little knowledge. I knew the basics, but the idea of eating all those saturated fats kind of scared me. I decided to get new blood tests every 6 weeks and compare the results to my older blood tests.

There are many competent medical clinics in Thailand. These clinics offer various blood tests at very reasonable prices. The blood test I most often get includes all the tests within CBC, Urine Analysis and Blood Chemistry. The cost of all these blood tests is only $15. Getting a blood test here every 6 weeks isn't too expensive. Get the number of blood tests that fit your budget.

Monitor your weight, your body fat percentage and your blood fat levels. You'll be pleasantly surprised.

Plateaus

It seems that any changes within your body that relate to LCHF occur in a series of plateaus rather than a straight downward slope. Changes like weight loss, lower body fat percentage, improved cognitive ability, increased libido, or any of the other benefits received through LCHF will occur, and then plateau.

An example of what I mean might be weight loss. With LCHF, you'll quickly lose weight then stabilize on a plateau before a second period of weight loss begins. Following that second period of weight loss, you'll reach a second plateau and again stabilize.

I can't present the science behind this, but can only relate to my own experiences and the experiences of my friends on LCHF. My guess is that a series of plateaus rather than a slope occurs because of the physical structure of our systems and cells.

There is a sort of *trick-plateau*, a plateau that reflects a change in body fat percentage rather than a change in body weight. After any significant weight loss, you'll plateau, your weight will remain constant. However, even though your weight is constant, your body will begin to change. You'll begin to lose fat and accumulate muscle. You'll do this without exercise.

I offer an example. While on LCHF, my weight dropped from 220 to 187 pounds. This change occurred in a series of plateaus. When I got to 187 pounds, I reached a plateau and stayed there. I'm there today. Every month, I look slimmer, but my weight remains about the same. What's happening? I'm losing fat and gaining muscle.

When in Thailand, I only where shorts, sandals and a polo shirt. It's quite rare for me to wear long pants. However, sometimes pants are a necessity. About 8 months ago, I purchased a new belt for my pants. I bought the belt at a market in Bangkok. The seller of the belt fitted the belt for me right at the point of purchase. He cut the leather until the belt fit perfectly. I wore the belt home, then promptly threw the belt in a drawer and forgot about it.

That was 8 months ago. Yesterday, I had to wear long pants and needed the belt. The belt was 3 inches too long. Even though my weight was constant, I'd lost so much visceral fat that my waist was 3 inches smaller. This is an example of the *trick-plateau*. There was no change in body weight, but a significant change in body shape.

Don't be afraid of these plateaus, with LCHF you'll lose weight or body fat. If you've been eating carbohydrates for a while, it may take some time to *retrain* your fat cells and the system regulating them. Don't give up, LCHF always works. Sometimes it takes a little longer for some than others.

Side Effects

It seems that some folks have side effects when they *begin* LCHF.

Potential Side Effects

- Headache
- Irritability
- Fatigue
- Dizziness

With LCHF you no longer eat carbohydrates. We've been taught to eat carbohydrates since we've been born. If your body is used to a lifetime of carbohydrates, it may rebel when they're taken away. I've read that some folks may need to ease their way into a low-carbohydrate way of eating, slightly reducing the number of carbohydrates they eat each day.

I didn't experience any side effects when I began LCHF. Most of my friends didn't experience any side effects when they began LCHF. However, I personally know of two cases of side effects.

Here's the first case. A few months back, I was in a pub in Thailand with a friend visiting from Washington State. My friend had lost 46 pounds using LCHF. He was very happy with his results, so we went to the pub to celebrate those results.

My friend's boss, the CEO of a very successful company, happened to be with us that evening and overheard our rejoicing. The CEO asked me specifics about his employee's weight loss. I summarized LCHF for the CEO, then suggested he give it a try. At a glance, I would guess the CEO needed to lose 50 pounds.

During the first two weeks on LCHF, the CEO suffered from *fatigue*. He was tired all the time. He toughed it out, and the fatigue subsided. He's now losing weight and feeling much better.

Here's the second case. Almost every Wednesday, I go to an elegant "gentleman's club" here in Thailand. I go on Wednesdays, because free sausages are available to the club's patrons on Wednesdays. Free sausages mean more customers. More customers mean more "hostesses." There are six types of sausages available: Cumberlands, chili, garlic, jumbo-hotdog, bangers and bratwurst. It's really quite a treat and LCHF friendly if you don't eat the buns.

The owner of this club is a great guy from California. I believe he's in his early 60s. The owner knew of my success with LCHF and asked me about it. I gave him the basics and asked for his email address. When I got home, I sent the club's owner a few chapters of this book. Eleven days later, I ran into the owner at my bank. He looked great. In eleven days, the club's owner had lost fourteen pounds. However, he did complain of a side effect. For the first seven days on LCHF, the owner had *headaches*. He toughed it out, then lost all that weight.

Hypoglycemia, low blood sugar: There is one potential side effect of great importance and that's the chance that a diabetic can experience *hypoglycemia*, low blood sugar. Diabetics normally take pharmaceutical insulin to reduce high blood sugar. A diabetic on LCHF won't have high blood sugar and the pharmaceutical insulin may drive blood sugar too low.

Note to Physicians

You're not going to like much of the content of this book. It's contrary to what you were taught in medical school. It's contrary to the medicine you currently practice. *Please, please, please try to keep an open mind.*

Put an obese patient or a patient with Type-2 diabetes on LCHF for one month. Tell the patient to eat when hunger is present and stop eating when hunger is satisfied. Tell the patient to satisfy hunger with saturated fats, not carbohydrates. Tell the patient to eat eggs, meat, fish and fowl. Tell the patient to eat green vegetables with melted butter, *not* margarine.

Choose a patient that will be honest with you about what was eaten and how the patient feels. Do your own mini-clinical-study. Get data both before and after. Compare the two sets of data. The results will blow you away.

"Detriments" of LCHF

Easily the biggest detriments of getting on the LCHF train are changes in energy and thinking. With LCHF, you suddenly have a lot more energy and your thinking greatly improves. How can those be detriments? They're detriments because you rarely feel like relaxing. When on LCHF, you end up zipping around all day, completing tasks, fixing things and problem solving anything that bothers you. Without those multiple spikes of insulin running through your bloodstream, you don't put things off. You don't feel much like relaxing.

One of the things I didn't put off was writing this book. I wrote 50,000 words in 5 weeks. It wasn't as bad as I'd expected. The real bitch was editing the book down to 40,000 words. That took 10 weeks. I rarely relaxed.

MORE LCHF

"LCHF applies to everyone."

The French Paradox

The French eat four times as much butter as we do. The French eat three times as much pork as we eat. The French eat 60% more cheese than we eat. The French eat a lot of saturated fats. The French also smoke twice as much as we smoke. *Yet, we have three times the amount of heart disease as the French.* That's the French Paradox.

Why are the French so lucky? Red wine? I call bullshit. It's because the French consume fewer carbohydrates than we do. The French don't drink soft drinks or eat breakfast cereal. The French satisfy their energy needs with saturated fats. Every *saucier* in France uses butter as a base.

Their cholesterol is higher because of the inflammation caused by their smoking. Their heart disease is lower because the cholesterol produced to fight the inflammation is the *right pattern* of cholesterol. Saturated fats satisfy their hunger as carbohydrates satisfy ours. After all, which country produces more fashion models?

LCHF vs. Other Diets

OK, LCHF sounds great, but how does it compare to other diets? Let's look at a few of the more popular diets.

The Pritikin Diet or "Whole Foods" Diet

This diet is medium-carbohydrate-low-fat. This diet allows you to only eat foods that are unprocessed or minimally processed, like fruits, vegetables, legumes, whole-grains, potatoes, lean meat and seafood. This diet encourages you to eat carbohydrates and stay away from saturated fats. "Whole-food" diets leave you hungry and cause inflammation. Go to the last few paragraphs of the chapter Advanced Discussion of Cholesterol to see a specific example on how "whole-food" diets affect inflammation and cholesterol.

Juicing

This diet is high-carbohydrate-no-fat. I'd experimented with juicing over the years with mixed results. I felt wonderful each time I juiced, but I never lost weight. Maybe I even gained a little. I'd be wired all day, then crash and burn.

I owned a large juicer while living in Costa Rica. I would often juice carrots and apples, carrots and celery, carrots and any vegetable odds and ends left in my refrigerator. Sometimes I would juice just plain carrots. One day a friend and I tried watermelon, celery and apple. We then went to the cinema. When the movie was finished, we both came down with projectile diarrhea. That was the last time I juiced.

The South Beach Diet
This diet is low-carbohydrate-medium-fat. I like this diet and had tried it several times with very good results. My only complaint about The South Beach Diet is that I couldn't sustain it. LCHF is much, much easier to sustain.

The South Beach Diet has you replace "bad" carbohydrates with "good" carbohydrates and "bad" fat with "good" fat, replacing foods containing *refined* carbohydrates, sugars and grains, with those foods containing *unrefined* carbohydrates, vegetables and limited whole grains.

You also replace foods containing trans-fats or saturated fats, vegetable oils and meat, with foods rich in monounsaturated fats or foods containing omega-3 fatty acid, olive oil and fish.

The primary difference between LCHF and The South Beach Diet is that LCHF encourages the consumption of saturated fats, while the South Beach Diet doesn't.

Years before I'd heard of LCHF, I would use The South Beach Diet to lose weight quickly. However, I'd always gain the weight back. I just couldn't keep at it.

I have a friend here in Thailand, a 57 year-old retired American from South Carolina. My friend was gaining weight every year, most of it around his stomach. Unaware of LCHF at the time, I suggested he try The South Beach Diet. He gave it a whirl and quickly lost weight. He removed the *refined* carbohydrates from his diet, soft drinks, desserts, pasta and bread, and began to take very long daily walks.

However, he begin to eat *non-refined* carbohydrates, whole grains in the form of muesli. He makes his own, mixing rolled oats and other grains with nuts and dried fruits. He's been eating and exercising this way for several years now and has lost a lot of weight. The guy looks great.

At my request, he recently sent me his blood test results. They were appalling. His daily consumption of grains has caused his LDL cholesterol to rise and his HDL cholesterol to drop to unhealthy levels. My friend looks pretty good, but his blood chemistry is pretty bad. Maybe he'll read this book.

The Atkins Diet

This diet is low-carbohydrate-medium-fat. This one's pretty close to LCHF and is a good diet. The Atkins Diet encourages you to stop eating carbohydrates and begin eating protein.

The primary difference between LCHF and the Atkins Diet is that LCHF encourages higher saturated fat consumption than Atkins.

The Paleolithic (*Caveman*) Diet

This diet is low-carbohydrate-medium-fat. This one's pretty good too. This diet tells you to only eat the foods that were available 10,000 years ago, fish, meat, vegetables, some fruits and nuts. You cannot eat grains, sugars and dairy products on this diet.

The primary difference between LCHF and the Paleolithic Diet is that LCHF allows for dairy and more fat to be consumed than the Paleolithic Diet.

Summary

Many of the above noted diets are what diets are traditionally thought to be, weight loss regimes intended for the short or medium term. They'll help you lose weight, but usually not keep it off without the presence of hunger.

With LCHF you simply replace carbohydrates with saturated fats. When you begin, you'll consume about the same number of calories as you did prior to going on LCHF. However, LCHF will *retrain* your system and cells, making your body efficient. You'll begin to consume fewer calories, but you won't be aware that you're doing so. It is this concept that that makes LCHF a *non-diet*. You eat whenever you're hungry. You simply won't be hungry very often.

LCHF & Children

This book is primarily directed at adults. Many of my anecdotes could be considered ribald. You may then ask, "But what about my children?" I hope to give you enough information so that you can make an *informed decision* about what to feed your children.

My next statement is a little strong. My next statement may even offend some of you: Every year our children are getting fatter, sicker and stupider.

Think I'm kidding? In the last 30 years, the percentage of obese children in America has tripled from 6% to 18%. In the last 30 years, Adult Onset Diabetes went from an *adult only* illness to an illness that now includes children. In the last 30 years, adolescent American children dropped to 28th place in mathematics and science as ranked against other industrialized nations.

Is it their fault? Is it their teachers' fault? Is it their parents' fault? Is it the government's fault? My answer is, "None of the above." It's because they eat too many carbohydrates and not enough saturated fats.

I'm childless, I made the profound decision of having a vasectomy at age 35. I live abroad, so the only American children I see are those on my return trips to the U.S., a few tourists and those children on American films and television shows.

I enjoy many American films and television series, but it always amazes me how American children are portrayed. Every adolescent film or television character is portrayed as complaining, lazy and needy. I thought it was just a matter of programming or a matter of too many pubescent hormones. I now believe that the programmers are doing their best to reflect actual American children.

We're raising a generation of children that are fat, lethargic and complacent. They don't play outdoors. They don't take menial jobs. They don't care about social issues. Their typical response to anything of consequence is, "Whatever." They think we owe them everything. They think they're entitled.

I thought they lacked character. I thought they lacked motivation. I thought they were spoiled little monsters. I thought these flaws were the flaws of their generation. I thought these flaws were their fault.

I was wrong. I now know that it's not their fault. It's what they eat that's at fault. American children consume huge amounts of carbohydrates every day. They no longer consume many saturated fats.

I'd like you to take a break from reading and walk into your kitchen. Open your cupboards and refrigerator door. How many carbohydrates do you see?

Carbohydrates cause the retention of fat, weight gain and insulin resistance. Is this what you really want for your children? Saturated fats help children think more clearly, solve problems more easily and become motivated to improve their lives.

You might have one of these problem children and don't know what to do. You've tried to teach, motivate and show love. However, you've hit that wall of rejection too many times. You've begun to give up.

Sit down with your child and try some simple questions. How does he or she feel? Is your child happy with his or her appearance, prospects or life?

Mother: Honey could I talk to you for a minute?

Daughter: Mom, I'm texting my friend.

Mother: Please, it's kind of important.

Daughter: Whatever.

Mother: As much as you don't want to believe me, I truly love you and only want the best for you. I want your life to be grand. I want you to be happy.

Daughter: [blank stare]

Mother: You know I've been on this crazy LCHF diet for two months now.

Daughter: [pause] Yes.

Mother: Well, the diet works. I've lost all kinds of weight and I feel a lot better. Haven't you noticed that I don't yell at you like I used to.

Daughter: Yeah ... but I thought that was because your doctor put you on some kinda new drug.

Mother: No, it's because I'm on LCHF. I don't eat carbohydrates any more. [pause] Do you think you might like to try it?

Daughter: [pause] What would I have to do?

Mother: You couldn't eat any more carbohydrates and that includes cereal, OJ, Coke, candy, snacks or even spaghetti.

Daughter: You've got to be kidding me. Mom, I'd starve!

Mother: No, that's not true. You can eat *anything* you want as long as it doesn't contain carbohydrates and you can eat *anytime* you're hungry.

Daughter: What *could* I eat?

Mother: For breakfast I'll make you bacon and eggs any way you like. For lunch you can have *two* hamburgers, as long as you don't eat the buns .... and NO fries. For dinner I'll cook you meatloaf, you always liked that, and broccoli. It always surprised me that you like broccoli. You can even add as much butter as you'd like.

Daughter: Really?

Mother: Yup. Eat all you want, whenever you want, but you can NEVER eat carbohydrates. Don't you want to be slim (again)? Try this and you'll lose 30 pounds and you won't ever be hungry. We could even do it together.

Daughter: [long pause] Mom, I really do love you.

Explain to your child what you've learned. Tell your child how LCHF has changed your life. You'll be surprised at your child's response. Your child wants to get better.

Try to put your child on a diet that replaces carbohydrates with saturated fats. It'll be tough, but explain that he or she won't be hungry and can eat whatever and whenever the child wants, just not carbohydrates. Try to get your child to do this for one week, then two, then three.

Once that time has gone by, again ask them for input. Is your child feeling better? Is your child happy with the weight loss? Is your child doing better in school? Are there things your child wants to try now?

The change in weight, mentality and motivation should be enough that your child no longer needs your input. Your child may even think it was his or her own idea. Maybe now you can get the lawn mowed.

Of course this means that you'll have to cook an omelet or bacon and eggs every morning instead of opening a cereal box. Better yet, teach your child how to cook ... and clean up.

LCHF & Exercise

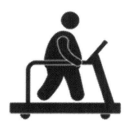

I believe that exercise, especially cardiovascular exercise, is damn good for you. If you have the means and will power, exercise once or twice a week. Exercise in conjunction with LCHF will improve your health and lower your weight faster than LCHF without exercise.

LCHF *will not* increase your muscle mass or give you muscle tone nearly as much as exercise. LCHF *will* reduce the amount of fat your body contains, but it will not replace that fat with very much muscle. With LCHF you'll lose the fat in your stomach, thighs and buttocks. With LCHF you'll lose the fat in your arms and legs. Without this fat, your arms and legs will become smaller and softer. The only way to really enlarge or firm up your arms and legs is through exercise.

Exercise isn't mandatory. LCHF will improve the lives of those people that don't exercise. Whether you exercise or not, you'll gain benefits from LCHF, better health, lower weight, higher energy and clearer thinking. However, only exercise will greatly increase muscle mass and improve muscle tone. Does masturbating count as exercise?

For many years my closest friend and mentor was David "Zigman" Zeigler. Dave was an athlete, very bright, very giving, very unconventional and a total head-case. Dave died a few years back of an aneurysm while riding his Harley in Guatemala. I love and miss this guy.

Dave's wife, Julia, is someone I set him up with in the late 1990s. I set him up because Julia blew me off every time I asked her out. If I couldn't have her, maybe my friend could. It worked out better than any of us would have imagined. Their marriage was one of those rare marriages. It worked. The three of us stayed close friends for many years. I love Julia as I loved Dave.

Following David's death, Julia began to workout hard almost every day. Julia is 44 years old, of Slavic-Polish heritage, and has the body and metabolism of a teenager.

Julia has a trainer, a big, bad Denver policeman. At her trainer's urging, she entered a sort of *boot-camp* competition. The competitors were to run around a circuit, stopping every few hundred meters and do an exercise, push-ups, sit-ups, chin-ups, etc. The competitors were to run the circuit three times. Julia was competing against all types of folks. Male high-school athletes, male bodybuilders, female workout fanatics. Badasses.

Julia crushed the field. She completed the full *three* circuits before any other competitor completed *two*. I think those 18 year-old football players she was competing against must have fallen in love with her right then and there.

I wanted to see how this much exercise affected cholesterol. I've repeatedly asked Julia to give me specific cholesterol results, but she never acquiesces. When I tell her of my grand success with LCHF, she *pooh-poohs* the results and reminds me that I lack true muscle tone. I'm not sure why she isn't pleased that I'm healthier and happier. Maybe it's because I've obtained these results without having to bust my ass at the gym 4 hours a day.

LCHF & Sex

If I were to make a graph of my libido, the graph would show a *shallow* downward slope from left to right. Not enough of a change to notice in the moment, but enough of a change to notice every few years.

I've always enjoyed sex. I've engaged in many sexual activities, both home and abroad. Activities that most Republicans would publicly condemn, yet privately condone. My mother often referred to me as a *letch*. I had to look the word up. My penis has dictated many of the major decisions in my life.

I moved to Costa Rica because *Ticas*, a non-derogatory name for Costa Rican women, are stunning, curvaceous and passionate. When I lived there, I had four *amigas-con-dereches (female* friends-with-benefits), two *latina* Nicaraguans and two *mulatta* Costa Ricans. Life was grand. I loved them all and they hated each other.

The only problem with *Ticas* is that they're very fertile and tend towards plumpness after the age of 22. Costa Ricans eat a lot of carbohydrates. Breakfast in Costa Rica is always *gallo pinto*, rice and beans. *Gallo* means rooster, denoting the early hour when breakfast is eaten, while *pinto* means two-colored, the white rice and contrasting black beans.

OK, let's get back to sex. In recent years, though I desired sex, that need, that overpowering need, was no longer present. I accepted this reduction in libido as part of getting older.

Then I began to eat LCHF. My libido quickly returned. My orgasms became more intense. My penis again began to dictate bad decisions. It was like turning the clock back a dozen years.

When I first moved to Thailand, a new pharmaceutical drug came on the market, Kamagra, a copy of Viagra, but in gel form. I was out carousing one evening and a friend suggested I try a Kamagra. I'd never used Kamagra, or even Viagra, so I thought, "What the hell."

Big mistake. I stayed out drinking, but never found appropriate company. It was a short night. I was going to play golf the following day. My usual golf partner was out of town, so he had a friend play in his place. I didn't own a car at the time, so the friend, someone I'd never met, offered to pick me up. He picked me up in a big pickup truck and off we went.

Well, you guessed it. The Kamagra in my blood stream along with the vibration of the truck produced the designed effect. I got a full erection. An erection you could hang laundry off of. Here I was, bouncing along in a pickup truck with a man I'd just met, a big, tough oil worker, and me with a full hard-on.

The guy was Canadian! Thank God he never noticed.

LCHF & Alcohol

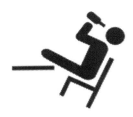

I may have a problem with alcohol. I'm out-on-the-town once or twice a week, often drinking way more than I should. Oddly, LCHF enables my semi-alcoholism. How? Because when I eat LCHF, I no longer have hangovers. That's right, one of the very *unexpected* benefits of eating and drinking LCHF, is that hangovers are a thing of the past. It probably has something to do with *Krebs Cycle* and *catabolism*, though I can only guess.

I've been abusing alcohol since puberty. Nights of wild partying were often followed by days of lying on the coach in a darkened, air-conditioned room watching anything on TV that didn't require much attention. Since I've reduced the carbohydrates in my diet, and removed them completely from the alcoholic drinks I consume, I *never* have any of those days.

Alcohol *does not* raise blood sugar. The Glycemic Index, how much a food is converted to blood sugar, of a vodka and soda is "0." I've switched to that drink now and haven't had a hangover since.

I have a private theory, a guess, that carbohydrates are a partial cause of hangovers. A beer contains about 13 grams of carbohydrates. Light beer about 6 grams. Wine, red or white, comes in around 5 grams per glass. Vodka has none.

I have a second private theory, another guess, that the reason you crave greasy, heavy foods following a night of drinking, is that your body is telling you it needs saturated fats to combat the carbohydrates in all of those Rum & Cokes running through your blood stream.

A little alcohol is beneficial to your health, actually raising your HDL. However, if you drink a lot, alcohol will inhibit weight loss. Here's a breakdown.

Alcohol

- Your body converts alcohol to fat in your liver.

- Your body burns the alcohol in your bloodstream before it burns fat or carbohydrates.

- Your body treats alcohol as a poison. Your liver will begin to work on it right away. Because it's busy, your liver won't regulate your *glucose* levels very well.

A glass or two of wine is fine. The carbohydrates in wine are fairly low. The same goes for light beer. If you drink more alcohol than you should, take vodka over ice or with club soda. Avoid mixing alcohol with anything containing sugar, soft drinks, fruit juices, tonic water, *sweet & sour* or energy drinks. Don't drink Jaegermeister, Goldschlager or Southern Comfort. These old acquaintances of mine are loaded with sugar.

LCHF & Smoking

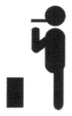

Smoking

Eating carbohydrates and smoking cigarettes is that deadly one-two punch that'll put you in an early grave. Smoking cigarettes inflames your arterial walls. Eating carbohydrates inflames your arterial walls. The inflammation caused by the combination of these two is compounded.

This compounded-inflammation really cranks up your body's production of LDL cholesterol. Because carbohydrates are in your bloodstream, the *wrong* pattern of LDL cholesterol is produced, the deadly Pattern B.

Smokers, fat or thin, will really benefit from LCHF. Why? Because though cigarette smoking results in inflammation and the subsequent production of cholesterol, it'll be the *right* pattern of cholesterol, the benevolent Pattern A.

Secondhand Smoking

I have a friend here in Thailand, an American from the state of Georgia. He's 74 years old and very fit. This guy is an enigma. He's a 14 handicap in golf. He's always full of energy and he has the libido of a teenager. He has a very beautiful live-in Thai girlfriend. The girlfriend takes very good care of my friend and has learned how to cook many American dishes. My friend loves baked goods. He loves pies and cookies, but what he really loves is cornbread. His girlfriend has learned to make them all.

My friend is neither a drinker nor a smoker. However, when he was much younger he was *married* to a heavy smoker. Last year he went in for a very thorough checkup and the doctors found some blockage, a lot of it. His red blood cells almost had to line up single-file to get through. It seems that his sweet tooth in conjunction with his prior exposure to second-hand-smoke gave my friend heart disease. He'd built up a lot of plaque, enough plaque that he had to have 4 stints put in place. He's alive and well, but the combination of carbohydrates and smoke almost ended a very fine life.

SATURATED FATS

"Saturated fats are good for us.
We've been misled for years."

Saturated Fats in Brief

We've been taught to avoid saturated fats, to limit the amount we consume. We've been taught that saturated fats lead to weight gain and heart disease. *We've been taught wrong.* Here's the breakdown.

Saturated fats

- Saturated fats raise HDL, good-cholesterol
- Saturated fats lower LDL, bad-cholesterol
- Saturated fats improve cognitive ability and focus
- Saturated fats reduce mood swings and depression
- Saturated fats increase a man's testosterone and a woman's estrogen
- Diets *without* saturated fats cause depression and disorientation
- Diets *without* saturated fats leave you grumpy and not much fun to be around
- Saturated fats are the good guys

Saturated fats are triglycerides that only contain saturated fatty acids. Foods that contain saturated fats are animal fats and some vegetables. Examples of animal fats that contain saturated fats are meat, butter and cream. Examples of vegetables that contain saturated fats are coconut oil and palm kernel oil.

There are three major types of fats, polyunsaturated fats, monounsaturated fats and saturated fats. Saturated fats are the best for you by far. No kidding. Many clinical studies have proved this. Your body needs saturated fats to survive.

The LCHF movement is really sweeping the Scandinavian countries. Scandinavians now require a lot of saturated fats. In late 2011, a Russian man was arrested for *butter smuggling*. He was arrested for trying to smuggle 90 *keys* (kilograms) of undeclared butter into Norway. Later that month, two Swedes were arrested for the same crime. They tried to smuggle 250 *keys* of butter into Norway. Maybe the *cartel* is behind this.

CARBOHYDRATES

"Carbohydrates are bad for us.
We've been misled for years."

Carbohydrates in Brief

We've been taught to consume low-fat carbohydrates, to include them in every meal. We've been taught that low-fat carbohydrates lead to weight loss and good health. *We've been taught wrong.* Here's the breakdown.

Carbohydrates

- Carbohydrates cause weight gain
- Carbohydrates cause low energy
- Carbohydrates cause arterial inflammation
- Carbohydrates probably cause many cancers
- Carbohydrates certainly cause childhood diabetes
- Carbohydrates are the single greatest cause of heart disease
- Carbohydrates are the bad guys

We've been misinformed for more than 50 years. We've been taught to believe that replacing bacon with oatmeal will lower our cholesterol. We've been taught to believe that drinking a tumbler full of orange juice is beneficial to our health. We've been taught to believe that eating unsweetened breakfast cereal is a way to lose weight. These beliefs are *fiction*.

Oatmeal, orange juice and breakfast cereal are carbohydrates. Eating them raises your blood sugar, inflames your blood vessels and locks down your fat cells. These are *facts*.

Carbohydrates & Evolution

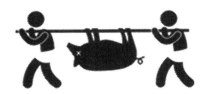

Carbohydrates are destructive. You shouldn't eat or drink them. Why are they so destructive? Because our bodies haven't *evolved* to process them. Human evolution is slow.

Human evolution is slow enough that our bodies assume we're living in prehistoric times. Our bodies assume the only foods available are meat and wild greens. Our bodies assume periods of famine are imminent. Our bodies assume that we're still *troglodytes,* prehistoric cave dwellers.

Agricultural evolution is much faster than human evolution. Agricultural evolution surpassed human evolution as early as 7,000 BC. It was then that we learned how to cultivate wheat and barley. It was then that we learned how to cultivate carbohydrates.

CAT scans of the 52 mummies stored in *The Museum of Egyptian Antiquities* showed that over half of the bodies showed signs of heart disease. How can that be? There were no fast-foods, trans-fats, cigarettes or Reality TV.

These folks got heart disease because whole-grains, carbohydrates, were the primary source of energy in their diet. The bodies of the Egyptians hadn't evolved enough to process carbohydrates and they got sick.

Like the bodies of the Egyptians, our bodies haven't evolved enough to process carbohydrates. Our bodies have only evolved enough to process meat and wild greens. Carbohydrates are a mystery to our bodies.

What happens when you consume carbohydrates? Your body thinks it has found a very rare, possibly once-in-a-lifetime source of energy. Your body knows that periods of famine are imminent, so your body locks that energy down.

Your body uses a complex system of receptors, enzymes and hormones to do this. It's your body's goal to store that rare amazing energy source, carbohydrates. Your body thinks the next famine is right around the corner.

Of course carbohydrates are no longer rare. They're everywhere. Take a stroll through your grocery store and try to determine which foods contain carbohydrates and which foods don't. My guess is that you'll see about 10 times as many foods high in carbohydrates as foods that aren't. Can you see why we have an obesity epidemic and why our children suddenly have Type 2 diabetes?

We're hard-wired to store energy. Why do you think we complete many meals with foods high in carbohydrates? Think this one through for a moment. Did you get it? Eating dessert is your body's way of telling your fat cells to lock down the energy you just consumed. We eat dessert to ensure that energy is stored.

Festivities like birthdays, weddings and anniversaries are all celebrated with foods high in carbohydrates, cakes, cookies and pies. We're celebrating the event with foods that will ensure that energy is stored.

We call one another names like *honey, sweetie, sweetheart, sugar, sugar pie, sugar-tits* and *sugar-britches,* terms of endearment synonymous with foods high in energy.

Carbohydrates are destructive because our bodies haven't yet evolved to process them. We crave carbohydrates because they're a great source of energy. An energy that's too often stored and not used.

DCA (Daily-Carbohydrate-Allotment)

How many carbohydrates are you allowed each day? I put a lot of thought into this question. I determined that the answer will be different for each person. To lose weight and improve health, each person will have his or her own "Daily-Carbohydrate-Allotment," their own "DCA."

Your Daily-Carbohydrate-Allotment, or your DCA, is the *maximum* number of carbohydrates that you can consume per day and expect to improve your health and lower your weight.

My DCA is about 80 grams per day. If I consume less than 80 grams of carbohydrates per day, I improve my health and I lower my weight. If I consume more than 80 grams of carbohydrates per day, I harm my health and add to my weight.

The greater the difference between the amount of carbohydrates you consume per day and your DCA, the greater the effects. If I consume only 30 grams of carbohydrates per day, my health quickly improves and my weight quickly drops. If I consume 300 grams of carbohydrates per day, my health quickly declines and my weight quickly increases. *The farther you eat beneath your DCA, the faster the results.*

How do you determine what your DCA is? Mostly through trial and error. Start by limiting your carbohydrate intake to 100 grams per day. Try this for a few weeks. Did you lose weight? Do you feel better? If not, lower the number to 80 grams per day and reevaluate.

Finding your DCA is much easier than it may seem. Your body will be aware that you're trying to help it. Your body will give you indicators when you're eating the right things. Your body will give you indicators when you're eating the wrong things.

I've observed that there are several factors that influence what a person's DCA is. Here's a list of those factors.

DCA Factors

- **Your exercise.** People that don't exercise have a lower DCA than those that do.

- **Your age.** The older you are, the lower your DCA.

- **Your gender.** Sadly women seem to have a lower DCA than men, especially post-menopausal women. Life is rarely fair.

- **Your ethnicity.** I'm not so sure about this factor. Statistics indicate that African Americans and Latin Americans are more likely to be obese than Anglican Americans. I believe that rather than *genetics,* it is the *foods* of those cultures that are at fault.

- **How long you've been overweight.** The *longer* you've been overweight, the lower your DCA.

- **How much excess weight you're carrying.** The more you're overweight, the lower your DCA.

- **How much visceral fat your body contains.** Visceral fat is the fat *between* your organs. The greater the amount of visceral fat your body contains, the lower your DCA. Visceral fat is more difficult to reduce in size than subcutaneous fat.

Review these factors before trying LCHF for the first time. These factors should help you determine your initial DCA.

I have a good friend here in Thailand, nicknamed "Quiet Larry." He's a Midwesterner of Teutonic background like myself. He's 68 years old, quiet, unassuming and a 6-handicap in golf. If you don't play golf, ask a friend who does what an incredible feat a 6-handicap is for a 68 year-old man.

"Quiet Larry" was pudgy, had high blood pressure and poor blood chemistry. Then I introduced him to LCHF. Following two months of LCHF, Larry's weight and blood pressure were the lowest in 30 years. However, his blood chemistry didn't improve very much. Not near the improvement that I'd experienced. I sat down with him and specifically reviewed what he was and was not eating. Larry was eating lots of meat, eggs and green vegetables. He wasn't eating very many carbohydrates. Why weren't his lipid profiles improving?

Then we found the culprit. "Quiet Larry" was consuming 5 or 6 light-beers every day. He said 5 or 6 light-beers, but my guess is that it's closer to 9 or 10. The carbohydrates in the light-beers pushed my friend over his DCA.

I went through a lot of acronyms before I settled on DCA. I looked at D-LIM, C-LIM, D-MAX, C-MAX, DC-Lim, DC-Max, Carb-Cutoff. Lots of acronyms. When I tried DCA, it felt very familiar. I wasn't sure why. Then I remembered. DCA are the initials of my long deceased father, Donald Charles Ahlswede. My father who died in 1980 at age 55 by eating too many carbohydrates.

Good Carbohydrates

I'm pretty tough on foods containing carbohydrates, especially foods containing *refined* carbohydrates. However, there are some foods containing carbohydrates that are good for you. Dark green vegetables.

Let's look at the carbohydrate content of a few. The quantities for all vegetables are 1 cup.

Dark Green Vegetables
- Broccoli = 12
- Asparagus = 8
- Spinach = 7
- Bok choy = 4
- Kale = 7
- Collard greens = 9
- Mustard greens = 3
- Swiss chard = 7
- Cabbage = 4
- Romaine lettuce = 2
- Iceberg lettuce = 2

Dark green vegetables are good for you, really good for you. They contain all kinds of fiber, vitamins, minerals and enzymes. Eat these vegetables with melted butter to add LCHF benefits. I often use thinly sliced Japanese cabbage *al dente* in place of pasta. It's pretty good with carbonara sauce.

Non-Green Vegetables
- Carrots = 12
- Potatoes = 32
- Corn = 41

Why bother?

A friend asked: "How do you like your vegetables?" I replied, "I like my vegetables the same way I like my women, dark, hot and covered in melted butter."

CARBOHYDRATES & WEIGHT

*"If you don't want to gain weight,
don't give your body a reason to make insulin."*

LCHF & Weight Change

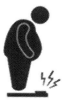

There are two schools of thought on weight change.

Old School

You're overweight because you're lazy and eat too much. You lose weight by exercising and eating less. This is what doctors have been telling us for *years*.

New School

You're overweight and lazy because you eat foods that make your body produce insulin. You lose weight by *not* eating foods that make your body produce insulin. You lose *even more* weight if you exercise. This is what doctors *should* be telling us. Most are reluctant to do so.

The reason behind weight change is that we're hard-wired to store energy as preparation for the next famine. When presented with a high-energy source like carbohydrates, our bodies go into a *store-energy-mode*.

Refined carbohydrates raise your blood sugar. To fight this high blood sugar, your pancreas produces insulin. This production of insulin causes your fat cells to *acquire* energy. This production of insulin prevents your fat cells from *releasing* energy. Here's the two-step science.

Insulin

- Step 1: Insulin causes your fat cells to *acquire* energy. More specifically, insulin stimulates greater *glucose* uptake by your fat cells. This energy is stored as *glycogen*, a long-term energy storage molecule.

- Step 2: Insulin prevents your fat cells from *releasing* energy. More specifically, insulin inhibits your pancreas from creating *glucagon*, the hormone that converts the stored *glycogen* back into *glucose*.

Think of insulin as a sideshow-barker for your fat cells, calling out to the *glucose* in your bloodstream. The *glucose* hears the barker's cry and enters your fat cells. Once the *glucose* enters the fat cells, the barker runs over and padlocks the door.

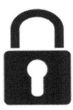

As you go throughout your day, your muscles demand energy. If you've eaten carbohydrates, your body produces insulin. This insulin makes your fat cells *acquire* energy. This insulin prevents your fat cells from *releasing* energy. You energy needs aren't met. You remain hungry. Your body tells you to eat again. This is *Old School* for "eating too much."

If you eat more carbohydrates, your body produces more insulin. This insulin makes your fat cells *acquire* more energy. This insulin prevents your fat cells from *releasing* stored energy. Your energy needs again aren't met. Your metabolism slows down. Your body tells you to rest. This is *Old School* for "being lazy."

Eating LCHF style, you consume very few carbohydrates. Your body doesn't produce much insulin. Your energy needs are met with saturated fats. Your body functions as it's been designed to function. Your body uses energy. Your body doesn't store energy.

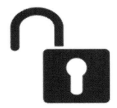

I return to the U.S. about once a year. It's on these trips that I noticed the weight change in many Americans. I even noticed the weight change in erotic film actresses. I hadn't seen an erotic film for some time, but viewed a couple during a recent trip to the U.S. Every actress was 20 pounds too heavy. Hell, if porn stars are getting fat, the obesity epidemic is for real.

Appetite-Controlling Hormones

This one's pretty recent, discovered about 10 years ago. It was discovered that your body produces chemical messengers classified as appetite-controlling hormones. One hormone is referred to as the Hunger Hormone. The other hormone is referred to as the Fullness Hormone.

The Hunger Hormone, *ghrelin*, is produced from cells in the wall of your stomach. *Ghrelin* is released when your stomach is empty. The Fullness Hormone, *leptin*, is produced from white-fat tissue. *Leptin* is released when your stomach is full. Both hormones enter your bloodstream and travel to your brain where they dictate your appetite and metabolism.

It seems that insulin impedes the effectiveness of these two appetite-controlling hormones. When you eat carbohydrates, your pancreas produces insulin. This insulin blocks much of the *ghrelin* and *leptin* from reaching your brain. When your stomach is empty, you'll be hungry, but not ravenous. When your stomach is no longer empty, you'll feel full, but not overly full. When you eat carbohydrates, you'll have a slow, steady stream of mild hunger that can never be satisfied.

With LCHF, your body doesn't produce much insulin. Your body won't block these appetite-controlling hormones. With LCHF, you'll feel hungry when your stomach is empty. With LCHF, you'll feel full when your stomach is full.

Types of Body Fat

Your body contains three types of fat.

Types of Fat

·   Subcutaneous fat, beneath the skin

·   Intramuscular fat, inside the muscles

·   Visceral fat, between the organs

Subcutaneous Fat

This is the soft body fat beneath your skin. Much of it is located on your thighs, buttocks and stomach.

After several months of coaxing, a close friend of mine, "M. Smith," from Washington State decided to try LCHF. "M" was one of those guys that had a *tire*, that roll of subcutaneous fat. Within three months of LCHF, he'd lost 40 pounds! "M's" *tire* is now flat.

This guy is one of the best friends in my life. He and I were roommates in the early 1980s, sharing a three-bedroom apartment in the East Bay of the San Francisco Bay Area. Our friendship continued over the years and he often visits me in Thailand.

"M" is bright, funny and very successful. He's 49 years old, drinks too much and smokes when he drinks. Before beginning LCHF, he suffered from health problems. His blood pressure was high, his blood chemistry terrible. He was on medication for both problems, often visiting his doctor.

Following three months of LCHF, "M" felt much better. He sat down with his doctor and explained how he'd lost the weight. He explained that he'd replaced the carbohydrates in his diet with saturated fats. His doctor was amazed. How could this patient lose weight and become so healthy by eating these "harmful" foods?

Luckily, this is one of those rare doctors who maintains an open mind. Hey, the doctor rides a Harley. The doctor believed the results to be accurate and related to LCHF. The doctor is now reducing "M's" intake of medication with the goal of eventually removing *all* medication.

Intramuscular Fat

This is the body fat that's inside your muscles.

Intramuscular fat increases the size of your arms and legs. How many times have you seen those heavy, lumbering, guys wearing sleeveless shirts showing off their huge biceps? Chances are those huge biceps contain muscle, but also contain a lot of intramuscular and subcutaneous fat.

To view an example of intramuscular fat, buy a well-marbled steak. All of those tasty ribbons of fat that you see in a rib eye are intramuscular fat. We pay extra for this type of fat. It takes grain containing carbohydrates to create this fat.

The Japanese produce some amazing beef. Kobe beef are cuts of beef from a specific breed of Japanese cattle renowned for its flavor. Kobe beef is well-marbled. Kobe beef contains intramuscular fat. This is accomplished by feeding the cattle grain fodder high in carbohydrates.

Contrary to popular belief, Kobe beef is not available in the U.S. American cattle ranchers have attempted to replicate Kobe beef by feeding their cattle beer, a food source high in carbohydrates. You don't want a body like a Kobe bull's, you want a body like Kobe Bryant's. Stop eating and drinking carbohydrates.

Visceral Fat
This is the body fat between your organs.

Many of the medical articles I've read state that visceral fat increases your risk of heart attack, stroke, dementia and diabetes. I think these articles are wrong. Carbohydrates, not visceral fat, increase your risk of heart attack, stroke, dementia and certainly diabetes. Enlarged visceral fat is a *symptom* of consuming carbohydrates. This symptom accompanies these ailments, but does not increase the risk of these ailments.

Before I began LCHF, I was getting heavier and larger every year. My stomach began to protrude. I'd often feel uncomfortable, full and bloated even though I hadn't eaten anything. My breathing was shallow and limited at times. What was happening to me? The probable cause of this discomfort was the accumulation of visceral fat pressing against the base of my lungs, stomach and other organs.

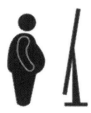

I often visit the beach in Thailand. It's about a five-minute drive from my home. The beaches are set up so that each patron is given a chair and umbrella. While seated, I can order a drink, a meal, a foot massage or pretty much anything that suits my fancy.

The beach that I frequent is often filled with tourists from different countries, Russia, Sweden, Denmark, Germany, England and Australia. Many of the German tourists are very big men wearing very small swimsuits. They have these cauldron-like bellies. They have these huge torsos supported by powerful legs. They don't appear to be flabby, yet their stomachs are immense.

You've seen this body type, that of a former athlete with no visible flab, yet a monstrous sphere of a stomach. Until I began to research the various types of body fat, I couldn't understand this. I thought, "How much do these guys eat?" I now know that it's not the stomach that composes this gigantic sphere, it's the visceral fat *behind* the stomach forcing it out.

I have two friends here in Thailand, one an American, the other a Canadian. Both are about 60 years old and both drink a lot of beer. They each have round basketball-like stomachs and oddly they each have protruding golf ball-like belly buttons.

It turns out that these *golf balls* are something called an umbilical hernia. This is primarily caused by intra-abdominal pressure. A pressure produced by the accumulation of visceral fat. It's that damn beer that's causing my friends to build up visceral fat and *pop* their belly buttons.

Sadly visceral fat is the toughest fat to remove. However, LCHF will steadily combat this demon. LCHF will begin to slowly act upon your visceral fat, shrinking it a little every month.

I'm a pretty hard drinker. I often consume too much alcohol. With alcohol in my diet, I steadily drop about 0.3 % of body fat per month with LCHF. When I began writing this book, I decided to cut my alcohol intake. I cut my hard drinking from 7 or 8 times a month to 1 or 2 times a month. With my limited alcohol intake, I dropped 2.1 % of body fat in one month. Most of it was probably visceral fat.

Order of Body Fat Loss

With LCHF, you'll lose body fat. That is, the fat cells within your body fat will release energy and become smaller. The loss of fat is in the following order.

Order of Loss

- **Subcutaneous Fat:** You'll lose this type of fat very quickly. This loss is noticeable and quickly apparent. You'll quickly drop off your *flab*. Your waistline, thighs and buttocks will quickly become smaller.

- **Intramuscular Fat:** Losing this type of fat takes a little longer. After a month or two of LCHF, you'll notice that your arms and legs are smaller in diameter. This isn't because LCHF causes a reduction in muscle mass. This is because LCHF causes a reduction of the fat *within* your muscles. Sadly, the only way to really enlarge your arms and legs without adding fat to them is to exercise.

- **Visceral Fat:** Losing this type of fat takes a longer time. It may take several months before you'll notice a big change in how far your stomach protrudes. Your waistline will quickly become smaller from the loss of subcutaneous fat, but the amount your stomach protrudes is dictated by the amount of visceral fat you're carrying around. Visceral fat is the most difficult type of fat to *evaluate*. You can accurately obtain your percentage of visceral fat and its location within your body through a CAT-Scan, but that's a bit pricey for most folks.

With LCHF you'll notice a *quick* change to subcutaneous fat, a *moderately quick* change to intramuscular fat and a *slow* change to visceral fat.

Fat Cells

The body of an adult human of average weight contains 20 to 30 billion fat cells. The body of an obese adult human may contain 80 to 300 billion fat cells.

It turns out that we're born with a specific number of fat cells. That number slowly increases until we reach puberty. The number then remains constant for the rest of our lives. There is an exception. The number of fat cells increases after *prolonged* obesity.

Our fat cells *enlarge and contract*. Fat cells are our storage units of energy. When we store energy, our fat cells enlarge. When that energy is released, our fat cells contract. If we consume carbohydrates, our fat cells are unable to release energy. The cells can still absorb energy, but the cells are restricted from releasing energy. If our fat cells become too engorged for too long, our bodies produce *more* fat cells. Hey, you've got to store the energy from that extra piece of carrot cake somewhere.

The Volume of Fat

You might like to know just how much fat you've lost in *volume*. Here are the calculations.

1 cubic centimeter of fat = 0.06 cubic inches

1 cubic centimeter of fat = 0.00198 pounds

1 pound of fat = 30.3 cubic inches (0.06 / 0.00198)

One 16 ounce soft-drink bottle = 31.1 cubic inches

One 16 ounce soft-drink bottle in volume = (about) 1 pound of fat in volume

Losing twelve pounds of fat would be like losing twelve 16 ounce bottles of fat.

Cans of Spam[11] would also be a good visual aid. You've all seen a can of Spam, that rectangular metal can about 3 inches tall and 4 inches wide. Well, each can of Spam contains 12 ounces. Four cans of Spam equals 48 ounces or three pounds. Four cans of Spam would be the same *volume* as three pounds of fat.

Spam Math

· Want to see what the 9 pounds of fat you lost look like? Line up 12 cans of Spam.

· Want to see what the 18 pounds of fat you lost look like? Line up 24 cans of Spam.

· Want to see what the 36 pounds of fat you lost look like? Line up 48 cans of Spam. I just realized that with LCHF, I've lost the equivalent of 48 cans of Spam.

---

11 www.hormelfoods.com/brands/spam/default.aspx

Oddly, Spam is a good LCHF food, containing only 6 grams of carbohydrates per *entire* can. I haven't had any Spam in years, but I have tasty memories of eating fried Spam and eggs after a night of heavy drinking.

If the *volume* of fat really intrigues you, go to Amazon and buy a *Five-Pound Fat Replica* for $84.95. The replica got great customer reviews.

CARBOHYDRATES & HEALTH

"Don't eat foods that contain sugar or
foods that your body converts to sugar."

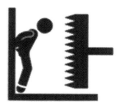

LCHF vs. Diabetes

LCHF fights diabetes. *Diabetes mellitus,* or diabetes for short, is the #7 killer in America with 70,000 deaths per year. OK, diabetes is only #7 in deaths per year, but how many Americans actually *suffer* from diabetes?

Diabetes in America

· 19,000,000 Americans are diagnosed with diabetes

· 7,000,000 are undiagnosed and most likely have diabetes

· 79,000,000 Americans are pre-diabetic

We are a nation with obscenely high blood sugar. Can you guess why? It's those damn carbohydrates!

It's having pancakes with syrup and a huge tumbler of OJ for breakfast. It's having a meatball sub and a large Coke for lunch. It's having spaghetti carbonara and garlic bread for dinner. It's having that midnight bowl of Rocky Road. It's having soft drinks, fruit juices, energy drinks, energy bars, cakes, cookies and candies all day long.

We eat the wrong foods. We eat carbohydrates. Carbohydrates are the reason people get diabetes.

Refined carbohydrates raise your blood sugar. To fight this high blood sugar, your pancreas produces insulin. This production of insulin causes your fat cells to *acquire* energy and be prevented from *releasing* energy. This production of insulin causes you to store energy and not use energy.

As you go throughout your day, your muscles demand energy. If insulin has padlocked your fat cells, you remain hungry. Your body tells you to eat again. If you eat more carbohydrates, your body produces even more insulin. The lock on your fat cells becomes even stronger. Your hunger isn't satisfied.

You remain in this endless loop of eating carbohydrates, producing insulin, locking down fat cells. Eating carbohydrates, producing insulin, locking down fat cells. On and on. This loop will cause your body to produce larger and larger amounts of insulin. This loop will burn out the receptors in your fat cells. Your fat cells will be unable to respond to the insulin produced. Your fat cells will be unable to absorb the glucose in your blood. *Your blood sugar will remain high.* That's diabetes.

Eating LCHF style, you consume very few carbohydrates and your body doesn't produce much insulin. Your energy needs are easily met with saturated fats. Your body functions as it's been designed to function.

LCHF vs. Obesity

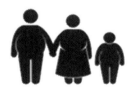

LCHF fights obesity. The medical community believes that many modern health problems are "obesity related."

"Obesity Related" Health Problems
- Heart disease
- Diabetes
- Cancer
- Arthritis
- Sleep apnea

What the hell does "obesity related" mean? Are they stating that obesity *causes* these modern health problems? It seems to be implied.

Obesity does not cause these modern health problems. Carbohydrates cause these modern health problems. Obesity is a *symptom* of eating too many carbohydrates. Obesity may occur at the same time as the health problems, but it does not cause these health problems.

Carbohydrates cause heart disease by making your body produce the wrong pattern of cholesterol. Carbohydrates cause diabetes by overloading your blood sugar control system. Carbohydrates cause cancer through inflammation at the cellular level. Carbohydrates cause sleep apnea by enlarging your fat cells so that your airway becomes blocked.

Obesity is a problem, a problem that's been growing every year. It's a problem that's growing in American and spreading worldwide. Carbohydrates are the cause of the obesity problem. If you're obese and no longer wish to be, get on LCHF. Stop eating carbohydrates and start eating saturated fats. It's really that simple.

LCHF vs. Inflammation

LCHF fights inflammation. We tend to think of inflammation as something that only happens to the *outside* of our body. When you get a thorn in your hand, the area surrounding the thorn becomes inflamed. You can both see and feel the inflammation.

Inflammation can also occur on the *inside* of your body. Many things cause *internal* inflammation, smoking, stress and carbohydrates being some of the most common.

Smoking is easy to understand. You introduce tar and nicotine into your blood stream. Tar and nicotine damages the interior of your blood vessels. They become inflamed.

The same is true for stress. Your body generates adrenaline during periods of stress. Adrenaline inflames the interior of you blood vessels.

What about carbohydrates? When you consume carbohydrates your blood sugar rises to toxic levels. This toxicity causes the interior of your blood vessels to become inflamed. Your pancreas produces the hormone insulin to reduce this toxicity. However, by then, the inflammation has already taken place.

Why do we care about inflammation? Chronic inflammation impedes healing. Chronic inflammation leads to heart disease. Chronic inflammation may be a precursor to cancer.

With LCHF, you don't eat many carbohydrates. With LCHF, your inflammation is reduced. With LCHF, your healing speed is increased. With LCHF, your chances of getting heart disease or cancer are reduced.

LCHF vs. Heart Disease

LCHF fights heart disease. This one's important. Heart disease is the #1 killer in the U.S. Heart disease takes the lives of about 600,000 Americans every year. LCHF reduces your risk of heart disease in two ways:

Reducing Risk

- Eating LCHF increases your HDL cholesterol. HDL cholesterol removes exhausted LDL cholesterol from your arterial walls.

- Eating LCHF allows for very few carbohydrates in your diet. Carbohydrates make your body produce the wrong pattern of cholesterol, a pattern that becomes oxidized as plaque.

Your body produces LDL cholesterol in response to the inflammation caused by eating carbohydrates. The LDL cholesterol fights inflammation by acting as a healing *salve*. When the cholesterol in this *salve* becomes exhausted, your body sends in HDL cholesterol to remove the exhausted cholesterol and return it to your liver to be recycled.

However, your body produces several types of LDL cholesterol, some good, some not so good. When carbohydrates are in your bloodstream, your body gets confused and produces the *wrong pattern* of LDL cholesterol. Let's look at LDL patterns. There are two main patterns of LDL cholesterol molecules, LDL Pattern A and LDL Pattern B.

Patterns of Cholesterol

- Pattern A is larger and more buoyant than Pattern B. Pattern A is associated with high levels of HDL and low levels of LDL and Triglycerides. Pattern A is *not* associated with heart disease. Pattern A is that healing *salve*.

- Pattern B is smaller and denser than Pattern A. Pattern B is associated with low levels of HDL and high levels of LDL and Triglycerides. Pattern B is associated with heart disease and the tendency towards Type 2 Diabetes.

- Pattern B get lodged in your arterial walls. Your body sends out white blood cells to *attack* these lodged particles. They become oxidized. These oxidized particles of cholesterol are known as plaque or heart disease.

This is how carbohydrates indirectly increase your risk of heart attack. They inflame your arterial walls causing your body to produce cholesterol. The wrong pattern of cholesterol is produced, a pattern that becomes plaque which leads to heart attacks.

Many doctors believe that genetics are the determining factor on whether a person produces Pattern A or B. I believe it is the amount of carbohydrates in a person's diet that determines whether a person produces Pattern A or B.

A special blood test called *polyacrylamide gradient gel electrophoresis* determines which pattern of LDL your body produces. I've been unable to find that test here in Thailand, though I hope to one day.

LCHF vs. Hypertension

LCHF fights hypertension. Hypertension, more commonly known as high-blood-pressure, can be a killer. Hypertension can cause stroke, heart failure or aneurysms.

Back in the mid-1970s, I served in the U.S. Navy as an HVAC engineer in charge of *A-Gang*. I worked on A/C, heating, hydraulics and pumps. This work helped me gain knowledge in *fluid dynamics*. I've used this knowledge to try to understand hypertension.

I believe hypertension is primarily due to the physical characteristics of blood vessels. The greater the resistance to blood flow or the greater the volume of blood pumped, the higher the blood pressure.

The formula for blood pressure would be "something like":

Volume of Blood Pumped x Resistance to Flow = Blood Pressure

If either volume or resistance is increased, pressure is increased.

Hypertension Questions

- What causes higher resistance? The buildup of plaque causes blood vessels to narrow resulting in higher resistance. Carbohydrates cause plaque buildup.

- What else causes higher resistance? Inflammation causes swelling resulting in higher resistance. Carbohydrates cause inflammation.

- What causes higher volume? Caffeine causes increased heart rate resulting in higher volume.

How about carbohydrates that contain caffeine? I'll take a Jolt Cola.

In the formula above, I say, "something like," because there are other factors, duration of *diastole* and *systole, venus pressure,* blood viscosity and the fact that your heart is not running at a constant speed.

LCHF vs. Cancer

LCHF fights cancer. For many years fats have been thought to be the cause of cancer. Clinical studies are now showing that *hyperglycemia*, high blood sugar, to be the cause of cancer.

Cancer

- Carbohydrates raise our blood sugar. Cancer cells use *glucose*, blood sugar, for rapid growth.

- Carbohydrates cause tumors to rapidly grow. Normal cells can use energy from *either* fat or carbohydrates. Cancerous cells *only* use energy from carbohydrates.

- Carbohydrates cause inflammation. Inflammation facilitates *metastasis*, the growth and spreading of cancer cells.

Smoking and being exposed to toxic chemicals inflames the delicate tissues of your lungs. That inflammation may lead to small-cell lung cancer. Chewing tobacco inflames the tissues of your cheek and gums. That inflammation may lead to mouth cancer. Carbohydrates inflame your arterial walls. That inflammation may lead to cancer or the growth of cancer.

Steve Jobs, cofounder and CEO of Apple, was diagnosed with cancer in 2003. He went on a high-carbohydrate-low-fat "whole-foods" vegan diet to cure this cancer. This diet caused his cancer to accelerate. The cancerous cells thrived on all the *glucose* produced by eating whole-grains. How could a guy so smart make such a stupid decision?

I have a female friend, Julia, who used to live in Roatan, Honduras, an island in the Caribbean. The medical facilities on the island were limited, so whenever she visited mainland Honduras, she'd get a full breast examination. I accompanied Julia on one of these trips.

We went to a local medical clinic where Julia knew the examining doctor. The doctor made the examination. Her breasts were in good health. They happen to be very lovely breasts. We invited the doctor to lunch and he accepted. As we three ate our lunch, I questioned the doctor on the presence of cancer in his patients.

He stated that he'd seen a dramatic rise in breast cancer in the past 7 or 8 years. He stated that he thought the growing number of breast cancer cases was associated with the growing number of fast-food restaurants.

I think the doctor *almost* got it right. I believe that his patients had increased their consumption of carbohydrates during those 7 or 8 years. This increase in carbohydrate consumption caused the increase in breast cancer. However, the patients may have bought those carbohydrates at fast-food restaurants or the patients may have bought those carbohydrates anywhere. There were simply more carbohydrates available during that period.

I have a very small family. Both of my parents had no siblings. I have no aunts, uncles or cousins. My father died of heart disease in 1980. My younger brother died in a motorcycle crash in 1981. My mother died of heart failure in 2004. My only living relatives are my younger sister, Ann, and her daughter, Kathy.

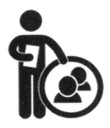

My niece Kathy graduated high school as a tall, slim, pretty, young woman. Then, she began eating a lot of fast-foods, eating and drinking a lot of carbohydrates. She got bigger and bigger, topping it off at 220 pounds.

At age 26, my niece was diagnosed with breast cancer. Kathy had a double-mastectomy to fight this cancer. Lots of surgery. Lots of chemotherapy. Luckily, she's in full remission and hasn't shown any sign of the cancer returning since 2007.

I strongly believe that it was those massive amounts of carbohydrates that she consumed that caused her weight gain and subsequent breast cancer. The inflammation resulting from that many carbohydrates was too much for the cells in her breasts to handle. The insult of inflammation was chronic, occurring every day. The cells finally rebelled and became cancerous. Who the hell gets breast cancer at age 26?

LCHF vs. Dementia

LCHF fights dementia. The website WebMD describes dementia as follows, "Dementia is the loss of mental functions such as thinking, memory, and reasoning that is severe enough to interfere with a person's daily functioning. Dementia is not a disease itself, but rather a group of symptoms that are caused by various diseases or conditions. Symptoms can also include changes in personality, mood, and behavior."

Got that?

Basically, dementia is a dramatic loss in the ability to think clearly beyond the loss one might normally expect from aging. The term dementia is derived from Latin meaning "without mind." For many years, the term was used to describe madness or mental instability. Dementia results from the destruction of *irreplaceable* brain cells. Chronic overindulgence of carbohydrates can lead to dementia.

Here's why. When you overindulge in carbohydrates, your body produces insulin. If your body produces too much insulin, you become *hypoglycemic* meaning your blood sugar is too low.

If you have several episodes of low blood sugar, you may cause damage to your brain cells. Patients taking pharmaceutical insulin are especially susceptible to *hypoglycemia.* With LCHF, your body will never produce too much insulin. You should never become diabetic requiring insulin injections. With LCHF, your odds of getting dementia are greatly reduced.

I first wrote, " ... your odds of becoming *demented* ... ," but that didn't really seem to work.

LCHF vs. Aging

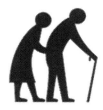

LCHF fights aging. Aging occurs when you use up your body's resources faster than it can regenerate those resources.

For many years I've held to the theory that if a substance speeds up your metabolism, it also speeds up the rate at which you age. The abusing substance is causing your resources to be used faster than those resources can be regenerated. Methamphetamine and cocaine are examples in the extreme. Caffeine and appetite suppressants are examples that aren't so extreme.

What about carbohydrates? Carbohydrates are *super-foods*. They're high in energy. They speed up your metabolism. Could it be true that eating carbohydrates accelerates aging? The logic is certainly there.

> *"The light that burns twice as bright burns half as long."*
>
> *- Dr. Eldon Tyrell in Blade Runner (1982), as played by Joe Turkel*

With LCHF, you reduce the number of carbohydrates you consume. Your body doesn't go into *high-gear*. You slow down your aging.

LCHF vs. Metabolic Syndrome

LCHF fights all the above. LCHF fights *metabolic syndrome*. This monster is the combination-plate of diseases. Metabolic syndrome, also known as insulin resistance syndrome, is a group of simultaneously occurring medical disorders or symptoms.

The *symptoms* that meet the criteria of metabolic syndrome vary depending on the source. Here's a list in total.

Symptoms

- Raised triglycerides (higher than 150)
- Raised blood pressure (higher than 140:90)
- Raised glucose levels after fasting (higher than 100)
- Raised C-Reactive Protein indicating inflammation
- Raised waist circumference (more than 40")
- Reduced HDL cholesterol (less than 40)

The *medical disorders* that meet the criteria of metabolic syndrome vary depending on the source. Here's a list in total.

Disorders

- Type 2 Diabetes
- Cardiovascular disease
- Hypertension
- Cancer
- Dyslipidemia
- Obesity
- Nonalcoholic fatty liver disease
- Polycystic ovarian syndrome
- Dementia

Metabolic syndrome is diagnosed as any *combination* of the above symptoms and disorders. Metabolic syndrome is caused by the *chronic consumption* of carbohydrates.

A friend of mine has medical disorders meeting the criteria of metabolic syndrome. He suffers from diabetes, high blood pressure, raised waist circumference and lowered HDL cholesterol. He's pretty unhealthy and he takes more medication than an obese radio talk show host.

I don't know how, but this guy just keeps on going. He leads a very full and active life. He has many friends and he loves the ladies. He's a pretty nice guy, just not very healthy.

LCHF Helps Healing

LCHF facilitates healing. I've had lower back pain for 30 years, I awoke every day sore and stiff and my golf swing was limited. My back pain was chronic, but tolerable. Then in 2010, the pain got worse. I could only sit for 20 minutes or stand for 10. My only position of comfort was flat on my back with a pillow beneath my knees.

I had to do something about the pain. I consulted a back surgeon at my local international hospital here in Thailand, Bangkok Pattaya Hospital[12]. The surgeon had x-rays taken of my lower back and later an MRI. Both showed that the disk between vertebrae L4 and L5 had collapsed causing a compression of the canal containing my spinal nerves.

He suggested I have corrective surgery, placing pins between the vertebrae to keep them separated and braces on either side of the vertebrae to keep my spinal column stable. I asked him when he could do the surgery. His reply, "Tomorrow, 6AM." Surprised at this early date, I agreed. I went home and collected my things. I returned and was checked into the hospital. I was given a *suite*, single occupancy.

Nurses and doctors ran tests on me throughout the day to determine if I was fit for surgery. Everything looked good. I spent the night in my suite and was awakened at 6AM. I was wheeled into the operating room and the doctors did their magic.

---

12 www.bangkokpattayahospital.com

I woke up around noon, only slightly sore. I spent the next 4 days convalescing in my suite, receiving service comparable to that of a 5-star hotel. The only thing lacking was the television programming. Thai TV programming is pretty bad, bad enough that the most watchable channel was Fox News. Thai TV uses Foley effects like Fox uses hyperbole. Hey, who am I to talk about hyperbole? This book is filled with it!

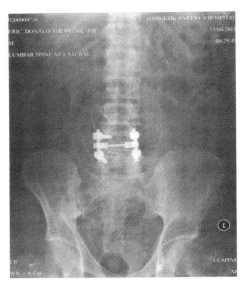

X-ray of the brace that was added.

During my stay, I tried to eat very few carbohydrates. At the time of the surgery, I'd already been on LCHF for 4 months. I didn't want to compromise the gains I'd made.

The day after I was released, I strapped on a Velcro back-brace and celebrated the last day of *Songkran*, the Thai New Year. Go to YouTube and do a search for "Songkran." The videos you'll find will amaze you. Thai New Year is one wild ride. The streets are filled with happy, mildly drunk people, foreign and domestic, all laughing and squirting water at one another. Though not in full form due to my very recent back surgery, I was able to participate.

My doctor was not pleased.

OK, what's the point of this story? The point is that LCHF enabled me to heal very, very quickly. I was 55 years old at the time, semi-alcoholic and reckless, yet I healed faster than any of my doctor's other patients.

Whenever I returned to his office for follow up x-rays, about every two weeks, my doctor would invite other staff members in to view my rapid recovery. He and the others would look at me in wonder. How could this crazy *farang* (foreigner) heal so quickly? Of course I held court. I explained that because I was eating LCHF, the inflammation resulting from the surgery was minimized. Minimal inflammation equals faster healing.

Though not related to LCHF, you may be wondering what my back surgery and those 5 days in a suite-like hospital room cost. Total cost was $12,000 of which my Thai insurance covered $11,000. I really do love this country.

My back pain is gone. The surgery worked. My back is in better shape today than it was 25 years ago.

If you're concerned about your own inflammation level, you might try a CRP (C-Reactive Protein) test. CRP is a protein found in your blood. The levels of CRP rise when inflammation is present. I recently had mine checked. My results were 0.111 mg/dL, the reference range was < 0.748 mg/dL. My inflammation is negligible.

If you're scheduled to have any kind of surgery, I strongly suggest you get on LCHF for the two months preceding the operation. Do this even if you decide not to use LCHF for any other reason.

LCHF Helps Bone Density

LCHF facilitates greater bone density. "Medical authorities" assumed that a diet low in carbohydrates would result in bone loss. They assumed this to be true because a low-carbohydrate diet would result in increased levels of calcium in the urine. It was assumed that this calcium had to come from bones.

Again, the "authorities" were wrong. Clinical studies have shown that diets low in carbohydrates and high in proteins result in *greater* bone density.

On one of my back surgery follow-up examinations, my doctor brought in the doctor that had assisted him. The second doctor commented on my miraculous healing. He also joked about how difficult it was to get the lag-screws holding the supporting bracket into place. He said, "Your bones too hard! Very strong. Very hard to work on."

I asked him if that was a bad thing. He answered, "Your bones very good, like bones of young man."

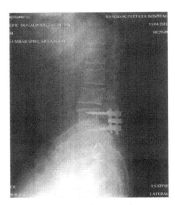

Look at the size of those lag-screws.

LCHF Helps General Health

LCHF may facilitate general health. There are hundreds of pharmacies and medical clinics in Thailand. All of them are very inexpensive. Both prescription and nonprescription drugs can be bought for a fraction of what they'd cost in the U.S.

Medical care is also inexpensive with a base fee of $15 for a visit to the doctor. It's easy and inexpensive to cure any minor illness contracted in Thailand. From the flu to a cold to the *clap*, it simply doesn't cost very much to fix. I've used both the clinics and pharmacies in Thailand many times with grand success.

Why am I telling you this? Because for the life of me, I can't remember the last time I was ill. I really don't remember having the flu or a cold since I began eating LCHF style.

The fact that I can't remember the last time I had a cold is not empirical evidence. I'm just sayin'.....

CARBOHYDRATES & CHOLESTEROL

"Saturated fats don't clog up your veins.
Carbohydrates clog up your veins."

Advanced Discussion of Cholesterol

Here are two statements of "common knowledge":

1. A Total Cholesterol count of higher than 200 means you're at risk for heart disease. A count of higher than 240 means you're at *high* risk for heart disease.

2. HDL is *good-cholesterol*. LDL is *bad-cholesterol*.

What do you think of these statements? Are they true or false, complete or incomplete, informative or misleading?

Total Cholesterol (TC) is calculated as follows:

TC = HDL + LDL + VLDL.

This is known as the Friedewald Equation. It was created by W. Friedewald in 1972. Almost every cholesterol test since 1972 uses this equation to calculate the *components* of Total Cholesterol.

Total Cholesterol (TC), High-Density Lipoprotein (HDL) and Triglyceride (TG) levels are *easy and inexpensive* to obtain. Low-Density Lipoprotein (LDL) and Very-Low-Density Lipoprotein (VLDL) levels are *difficult and expensive* to obtain. As such, LDL and VLDL are mathematically, rather than physically, obtained. The Friedewald Equation does this by estimating VLDL as 20% of TG. It then solves for LDL by rearranging the equation to LDL = TC − HDL − VLDL. This is a pretty clever way of using easy, inexpensive tests.

OK, enough arithmetic. Why do we care about the components of Total Cholesterol? Because we wish to determine the *ratios* of these components to one another.

Let's look at two fictitious test subjects.

- Subject A: HDL 30, LDL 100, TG 100. This subject's Total Cholesterol is 150. 30 + 100 + (20% of 100) = 150.

- Subject B: HDL 100, LDL 100, TG 100. This subject's Total Cholesterol is 220. 100 + 100 + (20% of 100) = 220.

Based upon "common knowledge," Subject A would be bragging to his coworkers of his miraculous "150"! Based upon "common knowledge," Subject B would be crying to his doctor of his dangerous "220"!

If you thought Subject A is healthier than Subject B, you'd be dead wrong.

Look at the test subjects again and compare their figures. Both test subjects have *identical* amounts of LDL and TG. However, Subject B has three times the amount of HDL, *good-cholesterol*, as Subject A. Even so, "common knowledge" dictates the he is the less healthy of the two. Subject B is considered the less healthy, because he has a higher Total Cholesterol count, a count that many insurance companies would have problems with.

Something is wrong with "common knowledge." Subject B is much healthier than Subject A. Why? Because his *ratios* are much better. With these ratios, Subject B is actually improving his health and removing heart disease.

In trying to understand this, I need to give you a little education into what cholesterol is and what it does.

One of the major reasons your body produces cholesterol is to combat the inflammation of blood vessels, primarily your arterial walls. Think of cholesterol as a salve that aids in the healing process. If your arterial walls are inflamed, your body tells your liver to produce cholesterol. Your body uses proteins called LDL (Low-Density Lipoproteins) and VLDL (Very-Low-Density Lipoproteins) to transport the cholesterol to the inflammation site to help with the repair. When the cholesterol becomes exhausted, your body sends in HDL (High-Density Lipoproteins) to transfer the exhausted cholesterol back to your liver for recycling.

This is why LDL is considered *bad* and HDL is considered *good*. One type adds layers to your arterial walls, while the other type removes the layers.

Of course *good* and *bad* are inaccurate. If your arterial walls are inflamed, your body knows to repair the inflammation. Your body uses LDL (carried) cholesterol to do so. Your body needs LDL and VLDL to repair itself, but it also needs HDL to remove the exhausted cholesterol from the repair site.

There are many ways to determine the risk of heart disease. Let's look at four ways using the figures from our test subjects.

Total Cholesterol

The most common number used to determine the risk of heart disease is Total Cholesterol.

·   Subject A: Total Cholesterol is 150.

·   Subject B: Total Cholesterol is 220.

Subject A is healthier, right? Wrong. Both subjects have *identical* LDL and VLDL, but Subject A has HDL of 30 while Subject B has HDL of 100. The difference in Total Cholesterol is due to the difference in HDL. This example easily illustrates that Total Cholesterol doesn't mean very much. It's the components that matter, not the *sum* of the components.

Ratio of Total Cholesterol to HDL

Another common number used to determine the risk of heart disease is the Ratio of Total Cholesterol to HDL. This is a much better way of determining risk than just looking at Total Cholesterol.

·   Subject A: TC-HDL ratio of 5-to-1 (150:30)

·   Subject B: TC-HDL ratio of 2.2-to-1 (220:100)

The lower the ratio, the healthier the subject is. This ratio easily illustrates that Subject B is the healthier of the two. The *American Heart Association* recommends a Total Cholesterol to HDL ratio of 5-to-1 or lower. With LCHF you'll easily obtain ratios far lower than that. Mine is usually 2.5-to-1.

HDL as a Percentage of Total Cholesterol

The above noted Ratio of Total Cholesterol to HDL is kind of clunky. A better way of using the data would be to view HDL as a *percentage* of Total Cholesterol. This calculation gives you a much better mental image. Think of it as a pie chart.

·   Subject A: HDL is 20% of TC (30/150)

·   Subject B: HDL is 45% of TC (100/220)

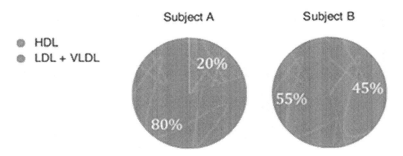

Subject A   Subject B

- HDL
- LDL + VLDL

Subject A: 20%, 80%

Subject B: 55%, 45%

These pie charts illustrate HDL as a percentage of Total Cholesterol.

Ratio of Low-Density to High-Density Lipids

There's yet another way of looking at these numbers. I believe that the ratio of (LDL + VLDL) to HDL is equally if not more important. Let's look at the ratio of the cholesterol doing the work, *low-density-lipids*, to the cholesterol cleaning up the work-site, *high-density-lipids*.

- Subject A: (LDL+VLDL)/HDL ratio of 4-to-1 (100+20:30)

- Subject B: (LDL+VLDL)/HDL ratio of 1.2-to-1 (100+20:100)

Your goal should be to raise your HDL and to lower your LDL and VLDL until HDL > LDL+VLDL. Eating LCHF will help you to achieve this goal. LCHF raises your HDL and lowers your LDL and VLDL. It's really that simple.

I first created the pie charts above to illustrate HDL as a Percentage of Total Cholesterol. However, these charts can also be applied to the Ratio of Low-Density to High-Density Lipids. In the Subject A chart, you can see that there's not enough *high-density-lipids* to clean up the exhausted *low-density-lipids*. In the Subject B chart, there's just about the right amount of blue *high-density-lipids* to clean up the exhausted yellow *low-density-lipids*.

There's a documentary entitled, *Forks Over Knives*. The movie explores a "whole food" way of eating, low fat "natural" foods and whole-grains. One test subject, the narrator of the movie, was overweight and had poor blood chemistry. He was placed on a "whole foods" diet for 13 weeks and his blood was again tested.

Here are his results after eating "whole foods" for 13 weeks: HDL 40, LDL 80, TG 169. His TC is 154. 40 + 80 + (20% of 169) = 154.

The test subject and his supporters were raving over the results. His Total Cholesterol was only "154"!

He's not as healthy as he believes. His ratios are:

TC/HDL ratio of 3.8-to-1 (154/40) HDL is only 26% of TC.

(LDL+VLDL)/HDL ratio is 2.8-to-1 (80+34)/40.

His body is sending a lot of cholesterol to combat the inflammation caused by his ingestion of whole-grain carbohydrates. Yet, there isn't enough HDL to remove the exhausted cholesterol from the inflammation site. His "whole foods" diet did improve his health, just not as much as LCHF might have. I bet the guy would have much preferred a T-bone instead of Tofu.

Rent this movie. It does have many valid points, but misses the point on saturated fats. You'll have to pause the movie quickly around 1:25:00 to view the final blood test results.

Improving your Cholesterol Profile

How to *raise* your HDL cholesterol

- Eat saturated fats. That's right. The consumption of saturated fats raises your HDL. I eat a lot of eggs, meat and heavy cream. My HDL is always about 100.

- Don't eat carbohydrates. Carbohydrates lower your HDL.

- Don't smoke. If you smoke, quit if you can. Quitting can raise your HDL by 10 points.

- Do drink alcohol, but only in moderation. One drink a day maximum for women. Two drinks a day maximum for men. These drinks will increase your HDL. Choose alcoholic drinks low in carbohydrates.

- Lose weight. For every 5 pounds you lose, your HDL should gain 1 point.

- Exercise. Aerobic exercise can increase your HDL by 5 points.

- Eat fish oil. Fish oils contain Omega-3 fatty acids, a substance that reduces inflammation and improves your LDL:HDL ratio.

· Take vitamin B3 (Niacin). This vitamin increases your HDL.

How to *lower* your LDL cholesterol

· Don't eat carbohydrates. Carbohydrates raise your LDL.

· Avoid stress. Stress creates inflammation leading to LDL production.

· Don't smoke. Smoking causes inflammation leading to LDL production.

· Sunshine. That's right. Exposure to sunshine causes your body to use up excess LDL cholesterol. Some of my best blood test results occurred right after spending a few days in the sun.

· Avoid anything that may cause inflammation. Inflammation leads to LDL production.

Cholesterol & Exercise

How does LCHF affect the blood chemistry of people who don't, won't or can't exercise? LCHF improves your blood chemistry, whether you exercise or not.

Here are two *real-life* examples:

Subject #1: 56 y/o, sedentary lifestyle, consumes too much alcohol, nonsmoker, Teutonic bloodline, family history of heart disease, Alzheimer's and *mitral valve prolapse* (bad check-valve in the heart).

After 12 months of LCHF eating, HDL 102, LDL 131, VLDL 20 (1/5 of TG 98). TC is 253 (102 + 131 + 20).

Subject #2: 43 y/o, daily strenuous workouts, consumes too much alcohol, former smoker, mixed bloodlines, family history of heart disease. Had minor heart attack at age 36 with severe constriction of arterial walls. Subject #2 smoked and ate carbohydrates at the time.

Following his minor heart attack, he was prescribed *statin*s as a way to reduce the risk of heart disease. After multiple years of low-carbohydrate eating and extreme workouts, HDL 65, LDL 92, VLDL 6 (1/5 of TG 32). His TC is 163 (65 + 92 + 6).

Subject #1 lives a life with too much alcohol and too little exercise.

Subject #2 is a workout fanatic and has been taking statins for a long time as a result of a very minor (is there such a thing) heart attack at a very early age.

#1's ratios are:

TC/HDL ratio of 2.5-to1 (253/102), HDL is about 40% of TC.

(LDL+VLDL)/HDL ratio of 1.6-to.1 (131+25)/102). For each one-point-six LDL plus VLDL he has one HDL.

#2's ratios are:

TC/HDL ratio of 2.5-to-1 (163/65), HDL is about 40% of TC.

(LDL+VLDL)/HDL ratio of 1.5-to.1 (92+6)/65). For each one-point-five LDL plus VLDL, he has one HDL.

Did you note that the ratios of these two subjects are almost identical? I suspect this to be true as both subjects eat few refined carbohydrates and many saturated fats. The reason #1's absolute figures are lower than #2's is probably due to his taking of statins.

This simple example is certainly not *evidence*. I used this example as an illustration. I do believe that even if you never wish to exercise, you can still dramatically improve your blood chemistry through LCHF. Many of my *non-exercising* friends eating LCHF have seen these dramatic improvements in blood chemistry.

Cholesterol Profiles of Friends on LCHF

A: 61 years old, very overweight, daily strenuous workouts, nondrinker, nonsmoker.

TC = 148
TG = 97
HDL = 42
LDL = 87

HDL is 41% of TC.

M: 43 years old, very active, physically fit, moderate drinker, nonsmoker.

TC = 163
TG = 65
HDL = 95
LDL = 32

HDL is 40% of TC.

C: 35 years old, athletic, physically fit, moderate drinker, moderate smoker.

TC = 202
TG = 128
HDL = 76
LDL = 98

HDL is 39% of TC.

M: 49 years old, sedentary, heavy drinker, moderate smoker.

TC = 165
TG = 143
HDL = 59
LDL = 67

HDL is 36% of TC.

E: 56 years old, sedentary, heavy drinker, nonsmoker.

TC = 248
TG = 110
HDL = 90
LDL = 136

HDL is 36% of TC.

L: 69 years old, moderately active, moderate drinker, nonsmoker.

TC = 230
TG = 114
HDL = 76
LDL = 131

HDL is 33% of TC.

All of these individuals are eating LCHF. As you can see exercise counts. Friend *A* with the highest HDL *percentage* is obese, but he's fighting *not* to be. He works his ass off every day and drops about 2 kilograms (4.4 pounds) per week.

Here's the cholesterol profile of a friend just *before* he began LCHF.

J: 62 years old, very active, physically fit, moderate drinker, nonsmoker.

TC = 238
TG = 116

HDL = 68
LDL = 147

HDL is 28% of TC.

Friend *J* had been on LCHF for 5 weeks at the time of this writing and is losing about 1 kilogram (2.2 pounds) per week. *Prior to trying LCHF,* he complained that his breathing often felt restricted. I told him that is was probably his visceral fat pressing against the bottom of his lungs. Since going on LCHF, his breathing never feels restricted. He's a *big ol' lug* and I love him as a brother.

Statins

Statins are drugs that lower cholesterol by reducing the effectiveness of an enzyme that plays a key role in the production of cholesterol. *Statins are the best-selling pharmaceutical drug in history.* There seems to be a fairly large debate on whether statins should be prescribed to those individuals who *do not* have cardiovascular disease.

Statins lower cholesterol, but have known side effects, particularly problems with the liver. A friend here in Thailand had been on statins for 10 years. The guy drinks some alcohol, but not over the top. At my urging he got a comprehensive blood test. His liver damage markers were very high, high enough that he stopped taking statins. His markers are now in line and because of his low-carbohydrate diet, his cholesterol is in great shape too.

Here are a few other potential side effects of statins; memory impairment, malfunction of the nerves, malfunction of the pancreas, malfunction of the liver and sexual dysfunction.

Using LCHF, your body will produce more HDL and less LDL. You won't need statins any longer. You won't have to chance these horrific side effects.

Insurance Company Guidelines

I wasn't surprised to find that life-insurance carriers have cholesterol guidelines. I'd always thought that they were pretty strict about Total Cholesterol levels.

It turns out that some carriers are now addressing Total Cholesterol-to-HDL ratios. Several use a 5:1 ratio, as the *American Heart Association* suggests, while others find 4.5:1 a better guideline for offering preferred rates. My current ratio is about 2.5:1 and I eat a lot of saturated fat. Hey, with LCHF, I can get better rates on term life-insurance.

FOOD

"If God hadn't wanted us to eat animals,
he wouldn't have made them so darn tasty!"
- Stephen Colbert,[13] I Am America[14]

Introduction to Food

OK, I've given you generalities about what to eat and what not to eat.

What to Eat and What Not to Eat

.   *Do* eat saturated fats.

.   *Don't* eat carbohydrates.

Now let's get specific. In this chapter, I'll be discussing specific foods, specific groups of foods and the preparation of foods. I'll define scientific terms and explain how to interpret scientific data.

Foods That I Eat

Foods that contain saturated fats are good for you. They also taste damn good. Saturated fats raise your HDL and increase the production of testosterone in men and the production of estrogen in women. Saturated fats help you think more clearly, solve problems more easily and keep your attention focused. I eat a lot of saturated fats. Here's what I normally eat.

Breakfast

For breakfast, I usually have 3 eggs fried in olive oil. If I decide to scramble the eggs, I may add some *unsweetened* whipping cream. I eat these eggs with a side of bacon or sausage. If I don't have any meat, I might add a half cup of chili or Bolognese sauce, then top it all off with a dollop of sour cream. I don't get hungry again for 4 or 5 hours. I don't get sleepy from eating these foods.

I eat a lot of eggs, some fried, some scrambled. When scrambling, I use little trick a short-order cook taught me. I add olive oil to the

---

13 www.colbertnation.com

14 shop.comedycentral.com/I-Am-America-And-So-Can/A/0446580503.htm

pan, then turn the heat up high. Once the oil is very hot, I pour the whisked eggs into the pan. Using the *tip* of a cooking spoon, I stir as fast as I can, trying to cover the entire cooking-surface of the pan. I stir until the eggs are cooked to my tastes, hard or soft. The eggs cook a lot faster than you'd think and always come out fluffy and perfectly done. Wish I could remember that old gal's name that taught me that trick. I'd thank her in my acknowledgments.

Lunch

For lunch, I may have a bowl of chili with sour cream and onions. I may have a pork chop with a side of spinach and melted butter. I may even have a bacon-cheeseburger with the top bun removed and a dark green salad with balsamic vinegar and olive oil. Again, I'm rarely hungry before 4 or 5 hours.

There were times when writing this book burnt me out. Yesterday was one of those times. I'd been editing for hours and was mentally beat up. I decided to do a little LCHF. I put 4 jumbo-sized eggs, diced onions and a *glug* of whipping cream into a bowl then whisked away. I scrambled the mixture in olive oil at high heat. Once done, I ate the whole mess in 3 minutes. Then it was back to editing, fully recharged.

Dinner

For dinner, I sometimes try to eat lightly, eating leftovers and a few pieces of fruit. At other times, I eat a little more.

One of my favorite dinners is ½ pound sirloin-beef bacon-cheeseburger with extra mayonnaise. The only thing is, I eat it with a knife and fork, buns removed.

As of the time of this writing, I'd just eaten a marinated rib-eye steak. I'd fried the steak in olive oil at medium-high heat. Just before the steak was done, I topped it with a couple of dabs of *bleu* cheese and added sliced onions to the pan. I ate the steak, onions and cheese followed by cantaloupe sprinkled with cinnamon. I slowly drank a glass of soft red wine with the meal. Between bites, I cleansed my palette with ice water mixed with lemon juice. I was satiated.

Beverages

I drink water with most of these meals and sometimes a Coke ZERO. I also drink *faux* lemonade. I fill a large tumbler with cold water, add a big squirt of lemon juice and a few artificial sweeteners. It's very thirst-quenching. At night I may have a glass or two of wine with my meal. If I'm eating thin-crust pizza or chili, I drink one or two light-beers. You can still drink carbohydrates while on LCHF, you just try to drink very few.

I have a low tolerance for caffeine. It hits me pretty hard. If I really want to get jacked up and speed through my day, I'll begin it with an LCHF coffee. I put one spoonful of premium coffee crystals into a cup, add two artificial sweeteners, fill the cup ¾ full of hot water and top it off with heavy *unsweetened* whipping cream. If I want a little variety, I slightly reduce the amount of coffee and add some soluble cocoa powder for a LCHF mocha.

Snacks

Throughout the day, I may snack on roasted almonds or cashews. I usually prepare my own, frying raw nuts in palm oil a couple times a month. If I've burned a lot of energy and become hungry, I often fry up a couple more eggs, maybe adding a slice of cheese.

When I'm hungry at night, I usually have a hot cocoa. I put a large spoonful of soluble cocoa into a coffee cup, add two artificial sweeteners, fill the cup up about ¾ full with hot water and fill the remaining quarter with heavy *unsweetened* whipping cream. I do miss the marshmallows.

I recently entertained a Thai woman at my home. It was getting late and I craved something sweet. I asked her if she'd like to share a cocoa with me. She didn't understand the word *cocoa,* so I tried *Ovaltine,* knowing that product was available in Thailand. She said yes to that and accompanied me to my kitchen. She watched as I performed my alchemy and sternly said, "This not Ovunteen!" I asked her to try it anyway. She did and said, "*Aroi mak mak.*" (very good tasting).

Thai Food

I also eat Thai food, a lot of it. Most Thai food is LCHF, as long as you skip the rice. I *don't* eat *Pad Thai*, the sweetened rice noodles found in most Thai restaurants in the U.S. It's kind of a touristy thing here and loaded with carbohydrates. I *don't* eat *Khao Pad Gui*, chicken fried rice. Too many carbohydrates.

I *do* eat a lot of *Pad Ma Muang Gui*, cashew chicken. I also like *Gang Garee Gui*, semi-spicy yellow curry chicken in coconut milk. I like *Kai Jeow Moo Sap*, a 3-egg omelet with ground pork in chili sauce. An American friend of mine on LCHF eats *Kai Jeow* with cheese. My all time favorite is *Pad Kaprow Mu*, spicy ground pork with basil served with a fried egg.

A neighbor of mine recently taught me how to make *Pad Kaprow Mu*. It's very easy. You add oil to a pan and get the pan very hot. Then add minced garlic and thinly sliced spicy, red Thai chilies. From there you add ground beef or pork, add a dash of sugar (I use Equal) and a little soy sauce. When all that gets done, you add the *Kaprow*, sliced basil leaves. Then stir, stir, stir. *Pad Kaprow Mu* is traditionally served over rice with a quick-fried egg on top.

The vapor produced from the frying garlic and chilies is very caustic. It's kind of like being pepper-sprayed. The kitchen at the bar I frequent, Tigglebitties, is directly in line with the bar. Occasionally the cook will make *Pad Kaprow Mu*. When she does, the vapors from the chilies roll down the bar and all of us foreigners are rubbing our eyes and cursing away. Thais love this stuff. *Pad Kaprow Mu* is to Thailand as a cheeseburger is to America.

Almost every grocery store in Thailand offers pre-made Thai sauces. The sauces come in pouches or cartons. The pouches contain paste to which you add water or coconut milk and then add the meat and vegetables. The cartons already contain the water or coconut milk, so only the meat and vegetables are added.

I often make *Gang Garee Gui* using these sauces. I get my pan hot and add a little olive oil. While the pan is heating I slice up a couple of raw chicken breasts and an onion, I add the chicken and onion to the pan, stir-fry for a bit, then add the contents of a *Roi Thai* brand carton of yellow curry sauce. The flavor of the sauce is a bit strong for my tastes, so I used to cut it with additional coconut milk. A friend of mine on LCHF makes the same dish, but rather than adding coconut milk, he suggested I add *unsweetened* whipping cream. I tried it his way. He was right. It was damn good.

Oddly the Thai people mostly use spoons to eat and cut. The use of a knife, fork or even chopsticks isn't common. When I first moved to Thailand, I took a young Thai woman to the beach where we ate all kinds of crazy things. She held her spoon in the air and seriously asked me, "You hab this one in Amelica?" She'd never seen a foreigner use anything but a fork.

The Thai people eat *fresh* food throughout their day. They rarely reheat things as Americans do. There are food-carts everywhere in Thailand. These food-carts are motorcycles with sidecars attached, containing cooking surfaces and a propane tank to do the cooking. I've never heard of one of the food-carts catching fire, but it surely must happen when putting an open cooking flame next to a 125cc motorcycle fuel system.

Except for rice, the Thai people eat LCHF. Their meals are usually of fish, meat and green vegetables with red-hot chilies. However, some Thais also love to eat insects.

I'm not kidding. Some Thais eat bugs. You can find a *bug-cart* on many blocks in the popular areas. The cart is bolted to a small motorcycle and features many small compartments displaying various types of arthropods, creatures with exoskeletons. I guess bugs might be considered LCHF.

Recurring Meals

At the beginning of the week I often make a crustless quiche, good for 5 or 6 breakfasts. Here's how to make it: Spray or wipe a meatloaf pan with olive oil, that amazing anti-inflammatory. In a bowl, mix 6 or 7 eggs, 1 cup or more of *unsweetened* whipping cream, a few dashes of Worcestershire and a few dashes of Tabasco. Add one package of frozen spinach, thawed and *wrung out* (important). I usually snip the wrung-out spinach into shreds over the bowl using a pair of scissors.

Mix thoroughly and pour into the pan. Top with a layer of cheese slices, then top with a layer of *raw* bacon. Bake the quiche for 1½ hours at 350 degrees or until an inserted knife comes out cleanly.

This stuff is good tasting and good for you, easily meeting the requirements of LCHF. Besides breakfast, I may have a slice of crustless quiche for dinner. It's great with a glass of red wine.

Once or twice a month, I treat myself to thin-crust pizza. A medium sized thin-crust pizza contains about 15 grams of carbohydrates per slice. I eat half of the pizza at the restaurant, 60 grams, and take the other half home, another 60 grams. That's still a lot of carbohydrates.

I've found that the best way to reheat the second half is by frying the slices in olive oil. You gain the anti-inflammatory benefit plus the added richness in flavor of the olive oil. I put a swirl of olive oil into a nonstick frying pan and set the heat to high. I add the pizza slices, crust down and cover them with a lid. Just before serving, I flip the slices over to warm them and crisp up the toppings and cheese. It's damn good this way, maybe even a little better than in the restaurant.

I'd lived in Thailand for 6 years before I found a really good pizza. The place is called *Drifters* and is located in Na Jomtien. It's a hole-in-the-wall owned by a Thai-Australian couple and located right on the very edge of the Gulf of Thailand.

When I lived in Costa Rica it took me 3 years before I found a quality pizza. The place is called *Cerros* and is located in the hills of Bello Horizante. Oddly the place is owned and operated by an Austrian.

Cerros produces the best pizza I've ever eaten. It took me a while, but I found their secret. Olive oil. The pizza is prepared in a very hot brick oven and just before serving, the cook tops the pizza with fresh herbs and a swirl of olive oil. Even back then my body recognized how good tasting and healthy olive oil is.

Holidays

I frequent a bar-restaurant here in Thailand with the incredibly poor name choice of *Tigglebitties Tavern* (an intentional reconstruction of *big ol' titties*). The customers all call the place *Tiggs* or *Tiggles*. It's an expat hangout owned and run by a great Thai-American couple, Nui and Randy. Most customers originate from the U.S., U.K., Australia and a few other countries. Their food is wonderful, the service perfect. I probably eat there 4 or 5 times a week.

The folks at Tiggles know I'm on a low-carbohydrate style of eating, so they willingly modify menu items. They might add an extra egg in place of whole-wheat toast. Maybe replace potatoes with vegetables or salad, that kind of thing.

There are two occasions where I eat quite a few carbohydrates, Thanksgiving and Christmas. Holidays I celebrate at *Tiggles*. The place is packed on these occasions. They serve a dinner of turkey and ham with sides of mashed potatoes, stuffing and jellied cranberry (the kind that retains the shape of the can). It seems as if everything is covered in smooth, delicious gravy. They also include a slice of either apple or pumpkin pie, topped with whipped cream. Because I'm such a regular, I'm usually given both. I cherish these two holidays because of these foods, taking my time and enjoying every bite.

I drink a few small glasses of red wine with the main course, but when dessert comes around, I order a cup of very black, bitter coffee. I take a small bite of pie, slowly savoring the flavor, swallow, then take a sip of bitter coffee to reboot my taste buds. Rinse and Repeat. I love these two *energy storing* holidays. I can make each meal last one full hour.

I attended a birthday party at Tiggles the night before I wrote the following paragraphs. The party was wonderful, free food, karaoke and lots of drinks. I hadn't been to Tiggles in the evening for several weeks. Everyone asked me why. I explained that I was cutting back on my alcohol intake and that I was writing an book. The American owner of the bar, Randy, asked me when the book would be available. I responded, "About 4 weeks." It then dawned on me that I hadn't written anything about Randy's weight change.

Randy shares the same birthday as me, October the 4th. He's exactly two years younger than me. Every year we have a party to celebrate our birthdays. This man is a friend of mine and I cherish his friendship. In recent years, I've watched him gain a lot of weight and harm his health. This guy took up smoking five years ago and put on 30 pounds. The combination of these two has put my friend's health in jeopardy. How did he gain so much weight so quickly? Probably from *drinking* too many carbohydrates. This guy buys his patrons a lot of drinks then the patrons reciprocate by buying him drinks. He likes to drink shots containing sugar, *B-52s*, *Girl-Scout Cookies, Jaeger-Bombs*, you know, girly-drinks. Never tease this guy about what he drinks though. He'll kick the crap out of you. He's become a little tub, but he's tough-as-nails.

Foods That You Eat (or used to)

If you're an American, chances are that you begin your day with breakfast cereal or oatmeal and honey. Or, you might have some whole-wheat toast with low-fat margarine. You might have some fruit or a low-fat yogurt. You'll probably have a glass of orange juice and a coffee. You think you're eating a healthy, light meal. Let's look at how many grams of carbohydrates these foods contain.

Breakfast
- One packet instant oatmeal = 36
- One tablespoon honey = 17
- One slice whole-wheat toast (no jam) = 13
- One glass (one cup) OJ = 25
- One cup coffee (unsweetened) = 0
- One yogurt, plain (8 oz.) = 17

Total = 108

Americans would consider this a very small meal. It's a meal that would leave most of them hungry.

Lunch
A small American lunch might be ham and cheese on whole-wheat bread with mayonnaise. Maybe you'll have a small bag of BBQ potato chips. As a treat, you might have a small chocolate pudding. Of course you'll wash this all down with a single can of Coca Cola.

- Two slices of whole-wheat bread = 24
- Ham = 0
- Cheese = 0
- Mayonnaise = 0
- One bag (1 oz.) BBQ potato chips = 15
- One small chocolate pudding (8 oz.) = 40
- One can (12 oz.) Coke Classic = 39

Total = 118

Even I'm hungry after thinking that's all I'm going to get to eat.

Dinner

How about spaghetti marinara with a large green salad and garlic bread for dinner? Have two glasses of red wine with the meal. Add a *sliver* of cheesecake with a decaffeinated coffee for dessert.

- Spaghetti (1 cup) = 44
- Marinara sauce (1/2 cup) = 18
- Garlic bread (3 small slices) = 48
- Green salad = 0
- Olive oil & balsamic vinegar = 6
- Red wine (2 small glasses) = 8
- Cheesecake (1/2 slice) = 10
- Decaffeinated coffee, unsweetened = 0

Total = 134

Snacks

You'll have to snack a little due to the small size of your meals. So, you have a Snickers bar during the day and a few cookies in the evening.

- One Snickers bar (2 oz.) = 36
- Three chocolate-chip cookies, soft-type = 24

Total = 60

Total for the entire day = 420 grams of carbohydrates

Wow!

Let's compare these foods to one packet of sugar.

One packet granulated sugar = 3 grams of carbohydrates

Now do the math. 420 / 3 = 140

These foods will have your body producing the same amount of insulin as eating 140 packets of sugar. Would you ever in your wildest dreams consider eating foods equivalent to 140 packets of sugar? You just did.

The meals I chose are simple and very small by American standards. Mentally review what you eat every day. How does it compare to this list?

Until I calculated the carbohydrates consumed in an American's typical day, experimenting with various meals, I had no idea that the figure would be that high.

I try to limit my carbohydrate intake to 80 grams per day. That's pretty far below the 420 grams in this example of small meals. The odd thing about LCHF is that it's so damn easy. You'd think that dropping from 420 grams to 80 grams would be difficult, but it's not. It's easy. With LCHF, your energy needs are always met and you never feel starved.

What's Good & What's Bad

·   It's not the pork sausage and eggs that are bad for you. It's the breakfast cereal, toast, hash browns and orange juice.

·   It's not the bacon-cheeseburger that's bad for you. It's the French fries, soft drink and hamburger bun.

·   It's not the beefsteak, butter and sour cream that's bad for you. It's the potato, rice and dinner roll.

·   It's not the butter fat in ice cream that's bad for you. It's the sugar in the ice cream.

Foods That I Miss

I really miss fruit juices. Sunday morning hangovers were often assuaged at IHOP. I'd order chicken-fried-steak, hash browns and a *full* carafe of orange juice. My mouth is watering as I write this. I really miss carrot juice, apple juice, cranberry juice and grapefruit juice.

I also miss baked goods. I would try to visit my sister Ann once a year and stay at her home in California. Ann would often surprise me with a pink cardboard box filled with *still-warm* breakfast pastries. I really miss those apple fritters. Ann and I would share one of those monsters and each have a cup of premium black unsweetened coffee to wash it down.

My friends miss carbohydrates too. Almost without exception, the food that my friends on LCHF miss is bread. Some of the guys miss potatoes, but they all miss bread.

The thing is, we don't miss carbohydrates as much as you'd think. The cravings are infrequent and never very strong. Saturated fats redirect our desires.

Cooking at Home

If you have the time, it's a lot easier to follow LCHF by cooking at home. A search of "LCHF recipes" on Google will provide you with many ways to prepare LCHF food. One site I stumbled upon is *Freckle's Food*[15]. I have no idea who Freckle is, but she provides some amazing LCHF recipes. Try her site. Try a similar search on YouTube for videos of LCHF food being prepared.

I recently came upon an amazing device that makes cooking LCHF much easier, the induction cooker.

In an induction cooker, a copper coil produces an oscillating magnetic field that induces an electric current *inside* the cooking vessel. These things are incredible. I put one of my high quality nonstick frying pans on the induction cooker. Turn on the cooker. Set the setting to *Fry*. I add a swirl of olive oil, then go get a carton of eggs from the refrigerator.

By the time I walk to and from the refrigerator, about 12 feet total, the oil is ready. It's very hot. I add the eggs to the hot oil and they immediately begin to cook. It's that fast, much faster than any conventional stove, whether electric or gas.

The unit I bought was only $40. They come in all sizes and wattages. I recently went to a birthday party at a bar I frequent, *Maam's Bar*. The folks there were using a huge, double induction cooker. The thing worked great. If you can afford one, try it. They're perfect for apartment or condo living or really any type of home.

Warning: Aluminum or copper pots and pans *don't* work on induction cookers as they're nonmagnetic. Most induction cookers

---

15 frecklesfood.blogspot.com

come with a pot made specifically for use with induction cooking. Most of the pots and pans you already own should work fine.

If you have an aluminum or copper pot and just have to use it, there's a workaround called an *induction interface disk*. The disk is heated by the induction cooker, which in turn heats the nonmagnetic pan. It's not nearly as efficient, but still workable.

Every pot and pan I already owned worked great with my induction cooker, especially the high-quality nonstick frying pans I'd bought when I began LCHF.

I have three Meyers Professional Choice frying pans in three different sizes. They're great. They all have very thick bases. They heat up fast, clean up fast and never show any wear even with repeated use. In recent years, the manufacturers of these pans have greatly improved the nonstick surfaces so that the surfaces are much more durable. All of my other cookware is gathering dust.

Cooking Oil

Olive Oil

Olive oil is mostly monounsaturated fat. It has been shown to be anti-inflammatory and may reduce blood pressure. It has been shown to reduce the oxidization of LDL cholesterol and helps prevent the formation of tumors. This is the good guy of cooking oils. I suggest you use it in place of any other oils.

I've tried to find health differences between the various types of olive oils, but they seem to be fairly equal. The various types do differ in flavor and color. The greener types containing more *chlorophyll* and *carotenoid,* resulting in a stronger flavor.

Olive oil is derived from a fruit, the olive, rather than a nut or seed as are most other oils. The health benefits of oils derived from fruits seem to outweigh the health benefits of oils derived from nuts.

Olive oil is stable in cooking and has a long shelf life. A great way to cook with olive oil is to add a tablespoon of real butter to the olive oil. The butter adds a ton of flavor while the olive oil prevents the butter from burning. My friend Laurice taught me that 25 years ago.

Coconut Oil

Coconut oil contains saturated fats. This oil raises your HDL *good-cholesterol*. This oil is very heat-stable, allowing it to be used in high-temperature cooking. It is slow to oxidize and has a long shelf life.

Palm and Palm Kernel Oil

Palm oil also contains saturated fats. This oil raises your HDL *good-cholesterol*. This oil is slow to oxidize and has a long shelf life.

I use palm oil in my deep-fat fryer to fry almonds and cashews. It took me a while to get the timing down, but I've got it now. I turn the deep-fat fryer on and set the temperature to the highest setting. It takes about 10 minutes for the oil to get there. I then add the raw nuts to the basket, lower the basket into the oil and let them cook for *exactly* one-minute-and-fifty-seconds. As the nuts fry, I stir them around with a metal spoon. I let the nuts cool, then put them into a bowl, add some Lawry's seasoning salt and a little crushed pepper. They taste great and keep well when refrigerated.

(Partially) Hydrogenated Vegetable Oils

These oils contain *trans fatty acids* commonly known as trans-fats. They may be labeled as hydrogenated vegetable oil, partially hydrogenated vegetable oil, vegetable shortening or margarine.

Partially hydrogenated vegetable is created by forcing high-pressure, high-temperature hydrogen gas into a vegetable oil thus changing the state of the oil from a liquid to a semisolid. When these semisolids are added to foods, the shelf-life of the food is greatly extended. These semisolids also improve the baking qualities of foods containing them.

In the late 1970s and early 1980s the Food and Drug Administration, World Health Organization, American Diabetic Association, American Heart Association, British National Health Service, Dietitians of Canada and the International College of Nutrition all warned of the dangers of eating coconut and palm oils. They suggested that oils containing trans-fats be substituted for coconut and palm oils.

Knuckleheads.

Don't be afraid to challenge the current positions of "medical authorities." They can get it wrong. They've got it wrong many times in the past. It wasn't too long ago that doctors endorsed smoking menthol cigarettes as a cure for chest colds.

Eating Out

If you're lucky enough to have a relationship with the people that work at the restaurants you frequent, they shouldn't mind adjusting what you order. They should be OK exchanging a food high in carbohydrates for a food that isn't. Potatoes for vegetables. French fries for salad. Toast for an extra egg.

If it's a restaurant you rarely visit, ask anyway. Most places here in Thailand don't mind. The only problem here is getting the information across. When you deviate from a specific menu item, the food you receive may be a little different from the food you ordered. Most of us just roll with it.

One of the wonderful and often frustrating things about the Thai people is their capacity for being polite. Almost every Thai I meet during my day is kind and polite. However, if there's a communication problem, they'll remain polite and say, "Yes sir." They'll say, "Yes sir" even if they have no idea what you've just said. It's more important for them to remain polite than to confront a misunderstanding. If you suspect that they haven't understood and try to explain further, a simple conversation often devolves into a *Who's on First* skit.

There are dozens of restaurants near my home, restaurants of all types; Thai of course, Italian, Russian, French, American steak houses and even Mexican.

One of my favorite types is Korean BBQ. These amazing places are clean, reasonably priced and very LCHF friendly. Korean BBQ costs a flat fee for all-you-can-eat. The price is about $6 for anything but seafood and $10 with seafood. You do have to pay for your beverages.

You take your seat, order your drinks and tell the waitress whether you'd like seafood. An employee, always a tough looking Thai man, shows up at your table with a thick ceramic pot containing red hot charcoal. He lowers the ceramic pot onto a steel cradle built into your table. The ceramic pot is topped with a steel cone. The cone somewhat resembles an inverted colander, with the sides sloping down into a circular water reservoir.

You head over to the many tables of raw food, the perishable foods protected by ice, and choose what you'd like to eat. I load up on raw pork, raw chicken and lots of green vegetables. LCHF at work here.

You return to your table where the BBQ cone is now screeching hot. You're given a small dish containing chunks of pork fat. Using chopsticks, you apply the pork fat to the sides of the cone to prevent sticking and add flavor.

You lay the raw meat onto the cone and add the raw vegetables into the water reservoir. As the meat cooks, some of the fat runs down the side of the cone into the water creating a sort of soup. Some of the fat drops through the holes in the cone to keep the charcoal raging hot.

You may return to the tables for more food at any time, experimenting with the different meats and vegetables. These places even have a dessert table and an ice cream station. It's a little tempting.

One time, I brought a few bouillon cubes, adding one to the water. The Thai woman I was with looked at me in wonder. She'd never seen such a thing, but was sure to bring a bouillon cube on her next visit.

Well, you try to arrange an evening like this with several people. You turn your food over and over and chat away. Everyone is cooking, chatting and drinking (low carbohydrate) beer. It's a hell of a lot of fun.

It's not difficult eating LCHF when you're eating out. A little knowledge and some friendly persuasion should help you fill your needs and avoid carbohydrates.

Breakfast Cereals

Most American children start their day off with breakfast cereal and milk. It's easy to prepare and it tastes damn good.

Let's look at how many carbohydrates these foods contain. The Nutrition Labeling and Education Act, or NLEA, suggested a serving size of ¾ of a cup for some cereals and 1 cup for others! Liars.

I've used the NLEA serving size for all cereals along with 1 cup of milk. Is this a lot? 1 cup of cereal combined with 1 cup of milk is just about the size of a major-league baseball, enough to fill a small bowl. Is this the amount of cereal and milk your kids are eating? I'd bet it's two or even three times that amount. Get out your measuring cup and try it. I did. Here are the carbohydrates in 1 cup of milk and the NLEA suggested serving sizes of breakfast cereals.

Milk:

- 1 cup 2% milk = 14

Choice of cereals *your kids* might eat:

- ¾ cup Cocoa Puffs = 23
- ¾ cup Cinnamon Toast Crunch = 25
- 1 cup Froot Loops = 26
- ¾ cup Cocoa Krispies = 27
- ¾ cup Frosted Flakes = 27
- 1 cup Lucky Charms = 29
- 1 cup Frankenberry = 29
- 1 cup Apple Jacks = 30

Choice of cereals *you* might eat:

- ¾ cup Special K Low-Carb = 14 (we have a winner)
- 1 cup Cheerios = 21
- 1 cup Special K = 22
- ¾ cup Wheaties 22
- ¾ cup Honey Nut Cheerios = 22
- ½ cup All-Bran = 23
- ¾ cup Bran Flakes = 24
- ¾ cup Honey Bunches of Oats = 25
- 1 cup TOTAL Raisin Bran 42
- 1 cup Healthy Choice Almond Crunch = 43 (not a very accurate name)
- 1 cup Raisin Bran = 45
- ½ cup Grape-Nuts 46
- 24 biscuits Frosted Mini-Wheats = 48 (I really miss these guys)

Sugar:

- 1 packet granulated sugar = 3

Some of the kid's cereals are healthier than ours!

Now double or triple the total based upon how many NLEA servings of cereal and the milk you think you or your kids might *really* be eating. Don't forget to add the carbohydrates in the sugar that they add to their cereal. Don't forget to add the carbohydrates in the OJ they drink.

Let's say your 12 year-old ate 3 cups of Lucky Charms with 2 cups of milk. He just consumed 115 grams of carbohydrates. That's equivalent to 38 packets of sugar. Your child's body will have to produce a lot of insulin to fight high blood sugar. This insulin will cause your child's body to *store* a lot of the energy from that breakfast cereal. If repeated enough, this insulin will burn out the receptors in your child's fat cells. Is it beginning to dawn on you why obesity and diabetes are now *childhood* diseases?

Some breakfast cereals are OK. You and your child can have ¾ cup of Special K Low-Carb and ¾ cup of skim milk for a total of 25 grams of carbohydrates. Or, you and your child can have steak and eggs with 0 grams of carbohydrates.

Pretty easy choice, don't you think so?

Soft Drinks

The energy in soft drinks is too concentrated. The energy in soft drinks is too easy to consume in quantity. Soft drinks are the major contributor to America's obesity problem. Soft drinks are the major contributor to America's diabetes problem. Soft drinks are the major contributor to America's heart disease problem. Our bodies are simply not designed to consume soft drinks.

We drink more and more soft drinks of larger and larger sizes every year. Here are the grams of carbohydrates in a soft drink you might order at a fast-food restaurant.

Coca Cola Classic:

- 1 Kid's Order = 31
- 1 Small Order = 41
- 1 Medium Order = 57
- 1 Large Order = 82
- 1 King-Sized Order = 108

103

Sprite:

- ·   1 Kid's Order = 30
- ·   1 Small Order = 40
- ·   1 Medium Order = 55
- ·   1 Large Order = 80
- ·   1 King-Sized Order = 105

Dr. Pepper:

- ·   1 Kid's Order = 30
- ·   1 Small Order = 40
- ·   1 Medium Order = 55
- ·   1 Large Order = 79
- ·   1 King-Sized Order = 104

Hi-C Orange Drink:

- ·   1 Kid's Order = 33
- ·   1 Small Order = 45
- ·   1 Medium Order = 64
- ·   1 Large Order = 94
- ·   1 King-Sized Order = 124

Now think about those *free refills*.

Let's go to 7-Eleven.

Gulp = 51

Big Gulp = 82

Super Gulp = 112

Double Gulp = 163

I try to limit my carbohydrates to 80 grams per day. I could drink a medium sized Coke and exceed that limit. This stuff is too high powered and contains too much energy to consume more than a sip. Soft drinks will screw your body up.

Several times a day, in both Central America and Thailand, I'd see those big red or blue soft drink trucks rumbling down the street, delivering their poison.

"The dealer for a nickel

Lord, will sell you lots of sweet dreams

Ah, but the pusher ruin your body"

- Steppenwolf "The Pusher"

Diet soft drinks are just fine. These drinks contain "0" carbohydrates. If you fear artificial sweeteners, first read the chapter entitled *Sweet Poison*.

Fruit Juices

When I explain LCHF to folks for the first time, they often give me an argument in favor of drinking fruit juices. Let's look at the number of carbohydrates contained in 1 cup of various fruit juices.

Fruit Juices
- Orange juice (from concentrate) = 25
- Orange juice (raw) = 26
- Apple juice (unsweetened) = 28
- Cranberry-Apple juice = 39
- Tomato juice = 10
- V8 Vegetable juice = 10

OK, fruit juices have fewer carbohydrates than soft drinks, especially tomato juice. However, it's pretty easy to drink more than one cup of fruit juice.

Beer

Tea and water are the only drinks in the world consumed more often than beer. Beer is made by *saccharification*, where starch is converted to sugar, and *ethanol fermentation*, where sugar is converted to alcohol. Beer is naturally sweet, so bitter hops are added for flavor and to offset the sweetness.

Beer contains carbohydrates. Let's look at a few of the more popular brands. All figures are the grams of carbohydrates in a 12-ounce serving, a typical can or bottle size.

Beer
- Budweiser = 10.6
- Bud Light = 6.6
- Bud Ice = 8.9

- Coors = 12.2
- Coors Light = 5.0
- Guinness Draught = 10.0
- Heineken = 11.3
- Heineken Light = 7.2
- Henry Weinhard's Amber = 14.0
- Michelob = 13.3
- Michelob Light = 6.7
- Miller MGD = 13.1
- Miller Lite = 3.2
- Molson Ice = 11.6
- Molson Light = 12.0 (can that be right)?
- Pabst Blue Ribbon = 12.0 (I drank gallons of this stuff in high school)
- Pete's Wicked Ale = 17.5
- Red Stripe = 13.8
- Sam Adams Lager = 18.8
- Sam Adams Light = 9.6
- Sierra Nevada Bigfoot = 30.3 (should be *Big-Carb*)

I must tell you that some of the values differed on the various websites I reviewed, but they were all pretty close to one another.

OK, we care about the number of carbohydrates, but there's a lot of information floating about concerning *maltose,* more commonly know as malt-sugar. The malted barley used to make beer creates malt-sugar, but this malt-sugar is used up during the fermentation process. There's no *maltose* in beer.

How many guys do you know that have *beer-bellies*? By now you've learned that a *beer-belly* is just the accumulation of visceral fat *behind* the stomach. If you have a *beer-belly* and want to get rid of it, try LCHF. Stop drinking beer altogether or at least switch to a beer with a very small number of carbohydrates. Then, greatly limit the number of beers you drink. If you can, switch to vodka and soda, no carbohydrates.

There's a great documentary entitled *How Beer Saved the World*[16]. Search YouTube or go to the website to watch this funny yet entertaining documentary. As you watch, think about the consequences of the carbohydrates contained in beer. Then, think about when and where heart disease first became a problem.

Halloween

All Hallows Evening, what everyone calls Halloween, is a holiday where children dress up in costumes and go door-to-door panhandling for carbohydrates.

Let's looks at some of the carbohydrates in the snacks given out. All sizes are *Fun Sizes,* smaller portions designed as treats. Why is smaller more fun?

Fun Sizes
·   Nestle's Crunch = 7
·   Kit Kat = 9
·   Tootsie Roll = 10
·   PayDay = 10
·   Snickers = 10
·   Reese's PBC = 10
·   Almond Joy = 10
·   Three Musketeers = 11
·   M&Ms = 12
·   Baby Ruth = 13
·   Butterfinger = 14
·   Tootsie Pops = 15
·   Skittles = 18
·   Candy Corn = 18 (this crap was always floating around loose in my Halloween bag)

They're all pretty even, around 10 grams of carbohydrates per tiny bar. How many bars do your kids *actually eat* on Halloween? Enough to put them into diabetic coma? Is Halloween a *gateway-carbohydrate* holiday?

---

16 topdocumentaryfilms.com/how-beer-saved-the-world/

"Healthy" Snacks

There are snacks being marketed as "healthy" that really aren't. These foods contain a lot of carbohydrates. Let's look at a few, but this time let's look at the carbohydrates *as a percentage of serving size*. The first figure is the grams of carbohydrates in a serving size. The second figure is the total grams in a serving size. The final figure is of carbohydrates *as a percentage of the total weight*.

"Healthy" Snacks

- Jello Pudding Snack, sugar-free = 13/106 = 12%
- Planter's Heart Healthy Mix = 5/28 = 18%
- Jello Pudding Snack, fat-free = 23/113 = 20%
- Healthy Choice Fudge Bar = 16/76 = 21%
- Fiber One Cereal Bar = 31/130 = 24%
- Bumble Bee Tuna Kit, fat-free = 24/99 = 24%
- Skinny Cow Cookies & Cream Bar = 20/63 = 32%
- Snack Wells Raisin Cereal Bar = 17/35 = 49%
- Redenbacher's Smart Pop = 22/35 = 63%
- South Beach Oatmeal Cookies = 16/24 = 67%
- Fig Newtons = 22/31 = 71%
- Triscuits, reduced fat = 23/29 = 79%

OK, some of these aren't too bad, especially the Jello Sugar-Free Pudding. The problem with these foods is that when you're eating them, you're eating carbohydrates. The manufacturers have to replace the "dangerous" fat with something else. That something else is usually carbohydrates. A second problem is serving size. No one I know can stop at the recommended serving size. So, double or triple the grams of carbohydrates in this data to see how many grams of carbohydrates you're *really* eating.

I've got to hand it to *Kraft Brands*[17] for producing a great informational site. You simply type in the food, click on the specific food and a perfect Nutritional Facts page comes up.

It should be noted that much of the information in this table was taken from the site, *FatSecret*[18]. This is a great site and will help you with LCHF.

---

17 www.kraftbrands.com/jello/products/pudding/pudding-snacks/

Years ago I held the position of Mortgage Officer. One of my clients applying for a mortgage was a sales representative for one of the larger food companies. Low-fat foods were the rage then, so I asked him about his sales of these items. He told me that the grocery stores located in the wealthier neighborhoods always bought a lot of low-fat products. He said that the grocery stores in the poorer neighborhoods *never* bought low-fat products. We then got into a discussion of the oils contained in preserved foods. He told me that *hydrogenated palm tree oil* was referred to in the food industry as *food lard*. Pretty insightful.

I've got a crazy friend, an American from Chicago named Billy. Billy works as an HVAC contractor in Afghanistan. He's a little younger than me and a lot bigger than me, especially around the middle. He's kind of like one of those Chicago parodies on SNL past. I enjoy this guy's company more than most. He truly makes me laugh.

Billy stops at Thailand once or twice a year for R&R. During his recent trip, we went to a BBQ at a mutual friend's house. I commented on his girth and asked him what he ate every day. He stated that the food was very bad in the compound where he works. To avoid the compound's food, he often snacked on things sent to him from the U.S. He has instant oatmeal and OJ for breakfast. He has tuna in water with a load of Triscuits for lunch or dinner. Carb-city.

I explained LCHF to Billy and told him the reason he was so heavy was that he was consuming too many carbohydrates. He was incredulous, "You mean that oatmeal and OJ are bad for me? What about my Triscuits? I go way out of my way to get them. I thought I was eating healthy!"

A few years back, Billy was visiting Thailand and asked to meet me for a drink. I drove to the destination, parked my car and walked to the outdoor bar we'd agreed upon. From a distance, I could see several bar patrons sitting and drinking. One of the patrons had long flowing blonde hair and was looking rather *Rubenesque*. I thought to myself, "Who's the blonde with the big tits?" As I got nearer, I could see that it was my pal from Chicago. I told him of my observation and he roared with laughter for 10 minutes.

Omaha Steaks

As this book neared completion, I sent my copyeditor and proofreader gifts of LCHF food. I sent them *Omaha Steaks*[19]. I'd heard of Omaha Steaks for years, but had never visited their site. I explored the site for a while, made some gift choices and had the steaks delivered.

While stumbling around on the site, I noticed that the *Omaha Steaks Nutrition Facts*[20] were available. I went to that tab and reviewed the information. If you can, try to open the PDF file at **omahasteaks.com/gifs/NutritionAnalysis.pdf** on your PC or Mac. Once the nutritional facts sheet is up, look for the *Carbohydrates (g)* column, a little to the right of center. Now focus on the numbers listed in this column and slowly scroll down the page. Try to pick out the higher numbers. Now look to the left to see which foods contain these higher numbers. All those wonderful steaks contain "0" carbohydrates. Yet, when potatoes, bread or pasta are part of the meal, the number of carbohydrates goes way up. What a great tool to illustrate the differences in LCHF and non-LCHF foods. Now look at the DESSERTS section. What the hell are *Lemon Lava Cakes* and why do they have 60 grams of carbohydrates?

Lean Cuisine

Lean Cuisine is a line of frozen meals marketed as low-fat versions of "normal" meals. The brand was first introduced in 1981 as a "healthier" version of Stouffer's products. They taste pretty good, are reasonably priced and have improved over the years. There are now over one-hundred Lean Cuisine meals.

I went to the website and found *Answers About Nutrition: Straight From the Nutritionists*[21]. This page included Q&A about sodium, but it also included a section on *Carbohydrates*. Look at the *Carbohydrate Questions (13 questions)*. You'll need to click on the icon preceding the *Q* to get the *A*. The answers they provided are definitely *old school*. Not in tune with LCHF.

Let's look at the Nutritional Facts of some Lean Cuisine foods, then compare those facts to its Stouffer's counterparts. I like

---

19 www.omahasteaks.com

20 www.omahasteaks.com/gifs/NutritionAnalysis.pdf

21 www.leancuisine.com/AsktheNutritionist/Index.aspx

Stouffer's and have wonderful memories of eating Stouffer's lasagna after a night of heavy drinking. Hell, let's try lasagna.

Lasagna
- Stouffer's Meat Lasagna (286 grams) = 39 grams of carbohydrates and 320 calories
- Lean Cuisine Meat Lasagna (286 grams) = 45 grams of carbohydrates and 320 calories

OK, maybe I chose the wrong product. Let's try another. Let's try meatloaf and whipped potatoes.

Meatloaf
- Stouffer's Meatloaf (263 grams) = 23 grams of carbohydrates and 300 calories
- Lean Cuisine Meatloaf (263 grams) = 25 grams of carbohydrates and 250 calories

About the same number of carbohydrates, but Lean Cuisine has 17% fewer calories. I guess that qualifies as "lean."

One more product, how about chicken pot pie.

Chicken Pot Pie
- Stouffer's Chicken Pot Pie (283 grams) = 64 grams of carbohydrates and 670 calories
- Lean Cuisine Chicken Pot Pie = DOES NOT EXIST

I guess even Lean Cuisine couldn't market anything with 670 calories as "lean."

Damn it, I couldn't resist one more, a food that I miss, fettuccine Alfredo.

Fettuccine Alfredo
- Stouffer's Fettuccine Alfredo (255 grams) = 42 grams of carbohydrates and 390 calories
- Lean Cuisine Fettuccine Alfredo (255 grams) = 54 grams of carbohydrates and 330 calories

These numbers are pretty telling. The serving sizes are identical. However, Stouffer's has more calories and fewer carbohydrates than Lean Cuisine. It appears that Lean Cuisine substituted carbohydrates for fat.

A lot of what I've just written may seem critical of Lean Cuisine, but I was surprised at how low the number of carbohydrates were in these foods. They're not too bad. By the way, I was ravenous after writing this section. All of these foods sounded very good right then.

Thais and Hot Dogs

Many of the Thai women I know are getting chubby. They're gaining a lot of subcutaneous fat. Most of them have noticed my weight loss and have asked me how I did it. I explain what I eat and what I don't eat. I suggest they try something similar. We then go through some lengthy translation issues as they make a detailed list of *yes* and *no* foods. Sometimes they're able to follow the list, but a typical response after a week of trying is, "I cannot do."

These gals work 12-14 hours a day and don't have time to prepare meals. I stumbled around and found a food they can easily and cheaply buy that fits LCHF. Hotdogs. There are thousands of 7-Elevens in Thailand. All of them offer hotdogs. Thais eat a lot of hotdogs. There's a major difference in the way Thais eat hotdogs and the way Americans eat hotdogs. Thais eat them with a sharp stick, *no* bun. Great for LCHF. Sliced hotdogs are bought in a clear, stiff, plastic bag. Condiments are added to the bag, then the pieces are eaten with thin, sharp sticks.

Thais also drink soft drinks differently than Americans. They drink them from a *bag*. It's not unusual to see a Thai holding his or her hand out like a pistol using their index and middle fingers to support a bag of Fanta while drinking through a straw.

I made a list of foods to eat and foods to avoid by using Google Translate. I circulated the list at the bars I frequent. Here's the flyer I wrote

น้ำหนักของคุณจะลงไปถ้าคุณทำเช่นนี้ **(Your weight will go down if you do this)**

เฉพาะกินอาหารเหล่านี้ **(Only eat these foods)**

เนื้อ **(Meat)**
ปลา **(Fish)**
ไส้กรอก **(Hot dogs)**
ผัก **(Vegetables)**

ไม่กินอาหารเหล่านี้ (**Do not eat these foods**)

ขนมปัง (**Bread**)
ก๋วยเตี๋ยว (**Noodles**)
มันฝรั่ง (**Potato**)
น้ำอัดลม (**Soft drinks**)
น้ำผลไม้ (**Fruit juices**)
ไอศกรีม (**Ice cream**)
ขนมหวาน (**Sweets**)

อย่ากินมากเกินไปของอาหารเหล่านี้ (**Do not eat too much of these foods**)

ข้าว (**Rice**)
ผลไม้ (**Fruit**)

คุณสามารถกินเมื่อคุณหิว (**You can eat when you are hungry**)
คุณหยุดกินเมื่อคุณไม่หิว (**You stop eating when you are not hungry**)

I had a little trouble with "Hot dogs." Every time I used Google Translate on "Hot dogs," I would end up with "Dog-hot," a warm canine. My Thai friend laughed when she read the Thai translation. She said, "This mean dog is hot, not hot dog."

Dental Care

If you're eating LCHF, you're probably eating a lot of meat. Not only is meat delicious, it improves your blood chemistry. However, the damn stuff gets stuck between your teeth. There's an easy solution to this minor problem. Buy a Waterpik.

Buy the best Waterpik you can afford and try it. Fill the reservoir with water and add a *glug* of mouthwash or hydrogen peroxide. Adjust the setting to your highest pain tolerance. Run the tip of the Waterpik along your gum line, inside and out, upper and lower. Repeat until the reservoir is near empty. You don't want to run the pump dry.

You'll be very surprised at the results. Your sink will be covered with bits of meat and tissue, even after flossing. You'll probably have some initial bleeding, but your gums will heal very quickly. The bleeding should no longer occur after only a few uses of the Waterpik. Your mouth will feel incredibly clean.

Bowel Movements

I'm pretty regular. I arise every morning and take care of business. This is a once-a-day business transaction. Since going on LCHF, my regularity continues. However, my feces and flatulence have become somewhat innocuous. LCHF seems to have diminished the level of foulness.

I've tried the *pull-my-finger* trick here in Thailand several times. The response is always the same. It's met with a blank, neutral *Billy Ray Valentine* look, displaying neither anger nor humor. My Mom used to fall for that old trick every few years. One time she even tried it on me.

One of the reasons I like living in Thailand is the *sai cet nam* or toilet-hose. Huh? Next to every toilet in Thailand is a short length of hose with a garden nozzle attached to one end and the other end connected to the toilet's water supply. Think I'm kidding? Do a Google search for "toilet hose," "bum gun" or "butt sprayer."

I love these things. Following my business, I simply bring the toilet-hose and nozzle to my rear, adjust the nozzle to the appropriate angle, relax and spray away. This device really washes me off. Much better than toilet paper. A 12-pack of toilet paper lasts me about one full year. If there's mud on your driveway, would you use a towel or a hose to clean it up? I'm so used to this device, that I feel unclean whenever I'm in a country that doesn't provide one. Of course the use of a toilet-hose in the U.S. doesn't take into account the frigid water supply of my home state, Wisconsin. Oh my.

Thais have very flexible bodies. It's not unusual to see a Thai squatting as a form of rest. Some of them even squat as they defecate. Here's an old joke: How do you know you're in Thailand? There're footprints on the toilet seat.

I knew a Thai friend who poops in this fashion. She'd have to lock the bathroom door though, because she knew I got a big kick out of seeing her perched on the toilet like a rooftop gargoyle. I'd be roaring away with laughter while she'd be screaming "Aaaaaaaaalllllleeeeeeek! Get out!"

FOOD SCIENCE

"Learn the components of foods.
Then, learn how those components affect your body."

Glycemic Index

The Glycemic Index (GI) is a measure of how much each gram of carbohydrates in a specific food raises blood sugar. The higher the GI, the more insulin your body needs to produce. This index uses *pure glucose* as a standard, with a Glycemic Index of 100.

The Glycemic Index of a specific food is as important as the number of carbohydrates a specific food contains. Most of this book focuses on the grams of carbohydrates in a food rather than the Glycemic Index of a food. The two really aren't that different. Foods with a high Glycemic Index contain a lot of carbohydrates.

Let's look at the Glycemic Index of some of the foods in a typical American diet.

Glycemic Index

- Grapefruit = 25
- Reduced-fat yogurt = 27
- Wheat tortilla = 30
- Ice cream (premium) = 37
- Spaghetti (whole wheat) = 37
- Apple = 38
- Tomato juice = 38
- Apple juice = 40
- Fettucini = 40
- Macaroni = 47
- Carrots = 47
- Grapefruit juice = 48
- Green peas = 48
- Potatoes (various types) = 50 to 85
- Orange juice = 50
- Banana = 51
- Corn tortilla = 52
- Snickers = 55

- Honey = 55
- Pita bread = 57
- Oatmeal = 58
- Coca Cola = 58
- Raisin bran = 61
- Ice cream (regular) = 61
- Spaghetti (white) = 61
- Raisins = 64
- Instant Oatmeal = 66
- Fanta = 68
- Cranberry juice (cocktail) = 68
- Special K = 69
- Rice cakes = 71
- Whole wheat bread = 71
- Watermelon = 72
- Popcorn = 72
- Bagel = 72
- Cream of Wheat = 74
- Corn flakes = 81
- Pretzels = 83
- Baguette = 95
- Fruit Roll-Ups = 99

Didn't some of these indexes surprise you. They certainly surprised me. How about pretzels vs. a Snickers bar? How about Fruit Roll-Ups?! Why would anyone feed his or her kid one of these?

You should try to avoid foods with a high Glycemic Index. Your body simply isn't equipped to process these super-foods. The Glycemic Index of most LCHF foods is less than 15. Eat LCHF.

There's a great website, *Self Nutrition Data*[22], that provides you with all sorts of information including something called *Estimated Glycemic Load*. This is a figure where the Glycemic Index is adjusted to incorporate serving size. The site also includes something called *Inflammation Factor*, how much a particular food

---

22 nutritiondata.self.com

inflames your blood vessels. Be sure to *always* adjust the serving size when looking up foods on this site. The default setting is often too high.

Glucose, Fructose and Sucrose

Glucose

Glucose is a carbohydrate. It is a simple sugar and is the source of energy for your cells. Glucose is also the source of energy for your brain.

Complex carbohydrates like wheat, oats and rice contain glucose. *Processed* grain products like breads, breakfast cereals, instant oatmeal and pastas often have *additional* glucose added to them. The glucose in complex carbohydrates quickly raises blood sugar.

Simple carbohydrates like fruits and vegetables contain glucose. *Processed* fruits and vegetables often have *additional* glucose added to them. The glucose in simple carbohydrates raises blood sugar but not as fast as the glucose in complex carbohydrates.

Fats like butter, olive oil and avocados are converted into glucose by your body. However, only about 10% of the fats consumed are converted. The glucose converted from fats raises blood sugar, but at a very, very slow rate.

Proteins like meat, fish and cheese are converted into glucose by your body. The glucose converted from proteins does not raise blood sugar as it is stored in the liver.

You need glucose to survive. You just don't need large amounts of it. Your body isn't designed to process large amounts of glucose. Large amounts of glucose are harmful to your body.

Fructose

Fructose is a carbohydrate. It is a simple sugar that is very sweet. Fructose is added to foods and drinks to make them taste better. Fructose is also added to foods to improve texture, stability and *browning*.

Grains like wheat, oats and rice *do not* contain fructose. *Processed* grain products like snacks, chips, breads, breakfast cereals, instant oatmeal and pastas often have *additional* fructose and glucose added to them. The fructose and glucose in processed grains quickly raises blood sugar.

Fruits and vegetables contain both fructose and glucose. *Processed* fruits and vegetables like jellies, jams and canned fruits often have *additional* fructose and glucose added to them. The fructose and glucose in processed fruits and vegetables quickly raises blood sugar.

Processed dairy products like plain yogurt, yogurt with added fruit, ice cream, sherbet, canned whipping cream and chocolate milk have additional fructose and glucose added to them. The fructose and glucose in processed dairy products quickly raises blood sugar.

Any food containing High-Fructose-Corn-Syrup contains fructose. Foods containing High-Fructose-Corn-Syrup quickly raise blood sugar.

You don't need fructose to survive. Your body isn't designed to process fructose. Fructose is harmful to your body.

Sucrose

Sucrose is a carbohydrate and organic compound. Sucrose contains the molecules of *both* glucose and fructose. Sucrose is the sugar that you use in your coffee and cooking. It doesn't matter if it's labeled as raw, white, brown or powdered, it's still sucrose and will quickly raise your blood sugar. You don't need sucrose to survive. Your body isn't designed to process sucrose. Sucrose is harmful to your body.

Trans-Fats

Trans-fats are unsaturated fats containing *trans-isomer fatty acids*. Trans-fats may be monounsaturated or polyunsaturated, but never saturated. Trans-Fats are the fats that cause inflammation and lead to LDL cholesterol production. Trans-fats damage your arterial walls. Foods containing trans-fats can include the following.

Foods Containing Trans-Fats

- Margarine
- Shortening
- Commercially prepared baked goods (donuts, cookies, pies)
- Commercially prepared snacks (crackers and chips)
- Baked goods mixes (cakes, cookies, biscuits)

- Breakfast cereals
- Energy bars
- Instant soups
- Candies
- Toppings
- Dips

Partially hydrogenated oil contains trans-fats. Avoid these oils and anything cooked in them.

Be careful with foods containing slightly less than 0.5 grams per serving. Look them up if you suspect this. The suggested serving size is often ridiculously small and even a small amount of trans-fats multiplied several times can produce harmful effects.

I decided to look up the trans-fats contained in fast-foods. The results surprised me. These folks still use too many carbohydrates, but they've reduced the amount of trans-fats.

You should avoid eating trans-fats as much as you should avoid eating carbohydrates.

Sugar Alcohols

When food manufacturers make something *sugar-free,* they often use sugar-alcohol in place of sugar. What the hell is sugar-alcohol? Sugar-alcohol is a hydrogenated-carbohydrate used to sweeten food. There are many sugar-alcohols. Here are a few of the more common sugar-alcohols. The number following the sugar-alcohol is the percentage of sweetness as compared to sugar.

Sugar Alcohols

- Xylitol = 100
- Maltitol = 90
- Erythritol = 70
- Mannitol = 60
- Sorbitol = 60
- Isomalt = 55
- Lactitol = 35

Sugar-alcohols are only partially digested. This means fewer calories and less tooth decay. Sugar-alcohols have a lower Glycemic Index than sugar. This means lower blood sugar.

However, sugar-alcohols are fermented in the intestines. This may mean bloating or diarrhea.

Because most sugar-alcohols aren't as sweet as sugar, more may be added to foods to achieve the same sweetness as sugar. This may result in only a minor change in the number of grams of carbohydrates consumed as compared to sugar.

I love living in Thailand, but I miss specialty products like sugar-free ice cream. I just couldn't find sugar-free ice cream anywhere in Thailand. Well, I recently had a big day. I found a place that will *make* sugar-free gelato. Gelato is Italian-style ice cream with less butterfat and air than American ice cream. The cost is very reasonable at $7 a kilogram, equal in volume to a little less than a half-gallon. I had a big grin on my face when I found this place. That is, until I checked the Nutritional Facts. It turns out that the manufacturer is using Maltitol as a sweetener. I had to dig into this. How many carbohydrates does Maltitol have as compared to a sugar?

Maltitol vs. Sugar

·   Sugar (1 tsp) = 4.2
·   Maltitol Crystals (1 tsp) = 2.0

Maltitol Crystals adjusted for sweetness = 2.0 x (100/90) = 2.2

Maltitol has about half the carbohydrates of sugar. Half is still too many carbohydrates. Also, Maltitol may cause bloating and diarrhea. I think I'll pass.

Sweet Poison

There's an email entitled *Sweet Poison*, originating in 1998, that circulates every few years. The email warns of the dangers associated with eating artificial sweeteners, particularly Aspartame. The email states that Aspartame may cause cancer, brain tumors and multiple sclerosis.

Like most *scare-emails*, it's a load of crap. Go to *Snopes*[23] to read a lengthy debunking of this email. Artificial sweeteners are fine. Any potential dangers associated with eating them are greatly outweighed by the dangers of eating carbohydrates.

---

23 www.snopes.com

I use artificial sweeteners. I use them to sweeten coffee and cocoa. I use them to replicate non-LCHF sauces and condiments. They work pretty well. Don't be afraid of using artificial sweeteners. Most of what you hear is just bullshit.

I have an American friend here in Thailand, 60 years old, 5'9" tall, physically active and one hell of a golfer. He possesses incredible touch and hand-eye coordination. My friend was an athlete in his youth, running marathons and participating in many sports.

My friend is now overweight, currently at 300 pounds. That's quite a bit for a guy only 5-foot-9. I think his all-time-high was 376 pounds. That high was a few years back. I remember him entering some kind of crazy bet with a bunch of overweight guys to see who could lose the *highest percentage* of weight. The stakes of the bet were fairly high. My friend blew everybody away. He went from 376 to 262 in 10 weeks. That's 114 pounds or a 30% loss. Amazing.

Sadly, he put most of the weight back on. Within two years, he was back up to 350 pounds. He would eat huge meals, drinking Coke after Coke with each meal. When he consumed alcohol, it was always Rum & Coke. I warned him that the primary cause of his obesity, though I never used the *O-Word*, was the consumption of these soft drinks. I told him to switch to soft drinks containing artificial sweeteners.

He told me that artificial sweeteners were too dangerous to consume. He cited the *Sweet Poison* email and some very ambiguous Yahoo article. Well, it took a while, but he finally gave up his sugary soft drinks. He now drinks club soda. It was a nice compromise.

He's changed his way of eating. He no longer eats many carbohydrates. He's begun to walk every day and begun to exercise. LCHF, walking and exercise has helped him lose 50 pounds. His golf handicap is dropping too. I like this guy a lot. I consider him a good friend. Watching him *permanently* lose this weight is very pleasing.

The Sneaky Carbohydrate

High-fructose-corn-syrup, HFCS, is produced from corn using enzymatic processing converting its glucose to fructose. This S.O.B. is in everything. It's in drinks, breakfast cereals, yogurts, condiments and many other foods.

Detractors of high-fructose corn syrup claim that the stuff interferes with appetite functions and is much more harmful than sugar. To me that's like saying arsenic is more harmful than strychnine. Who cares? I'm not going to eat either one.

There's a lot of discussion in the medical community concerning HFCS. It's been said that HFCS may lead to obesity, cardiovascular disease, fatty liver and diabetes.

The reason I'm bringing up HFCS is that if you decide to get serious about LCHF, you may begin to read nutritional information labels. Watch out for this guy. He can really screw your body up.

The Men Who Made Us Fat

There's a great documentary series entitled *The Men Who Made Us Fat (2012)*[24]. You can find it on YouTube or go directly to the BBC site. This documentary is wonderful, focusing on the effects of high-fructose-corn-syrup. I disagree with quite a few of the conclusions that were drawn, but it's a great watch.

King Corn

King Corn (2007) is a fascinating documentary about two East Coast friends who decide to farm an acre of corn in Iowa. The friends follow their corn, at least metaphorically, from the acre they'd planted to cattle feed lots and corn syrup production plants. Pay close attention to the portion of the movie dealing with the corn-fed cattle. Observe the health and weight of the cattle after being fed carbohydrates for the 5 months preceding slaughter. Try to apply what you've learned to what you're eating. *You can watch King Corn*[25] *on Hulu*. Sadly *Hulu* is only available for those viewers within the U.S.

---

24 www.bbc.co.uk/programmes/b01k0fs0
25 www.hulu.com/watch/255609/

NLEA

NLEA is an acronym for the *Nutrition Labeling and Education Act of 1990*. This act is responsible for those neat, concise labels you find on most food products. The NLEA is a U.S. Federal Law. Nutritional Fact labeling is *mandatory*. Guess who signed the act into law? President George Bush. That's "H.W.," not "W."

The law gives the Food and Drug Administration the power to require labeling on foods that are regulated by that agency. It *does not* apply to foods served at "normal" restaurants. The law also mandates that nutritional claims and health claims meet FDA regulations. Of course in recent years, many of the major food companies have begun to hire ex-FDA personnel. There might be a conflict of interest there.

With LCHF, you'll begin to understand what the facts on a Nutritional Facts label mean. You'll note how many grams of carbohydrates, sugars and trans-fats a specific food contains.

Here's an example of a Nutrition Facts label meeting the requirements of the NLEA. The food is a *Classic Cinnabon Roll*.

Nutrition Facts

Serving Size 1 roll

Amount Per Serving

Calories 880   Calories from Fat 320

	% Daily Values*
Total Fat 36g	55%
Saturated Fat 17g	85%
Cholesterol 20mg	7%
Sodium 830mg	35%
Total Carbohydrate 127g	42%
Dietary Fiber 2g	8%
Sugars 59g	
Protein 13g	

Vitamin A -	●	Vitamin C -
Calcium -	●	Iron -

* Percent Daily Values are based on a 2000 calorie diet. Your daily values may be higher or lower depending on your calorie needs.

One Cinnabon.

Let's break down the information. First check the *Serving Size*. Be prepared to do mathematics if you're going to eat more or less than the size presented. In this case, the *Serving Size* is *1 roll*. So, if you're only going to eat 1/2 of a roll, *divide* the pertinent information by two. If you plan on eating two of these monsters (is that even possible), *multiply* the information by two. Look at the *Calories* of this beast, 880 calories. Eating two of them would be consuming 1,760 calories!

Next look at the *Total Carbohydrate*, in this case, 127 grams. Eating two of them would be consuming 254 grams of carbohydrate, an amount equal to what I consume in a full week. Ignore the right-hand column, *% of Daily Values*. The figures really have no meaning as the recommended daily amounts are much too high. Our example shows 127 grams of carbohydrates as 42% of the recommended daily consumption. That means these knuckleheads are recommending you consume 300 grams of carbohydrates *per day* (127 / .42).

Let's do a second analysis, that of a single McDonald's cheeseburger.

Nutrition Facts

Serving Size 1 burger (114g)

Amount Per Serving

Calories 300   Calories from Fat 110

	% Daily Values*
Total Fat 12g	18%
Saturated Fat 6g	30%
Trans Fat 0.4g	
Cholesterol 35mg	12%
Sodium 750mg	31%
Total Carbohydrate 33g	11%
Dietary Fiber 2g	8%
Sugars 7g	
Protein 15g	

Vitamin A 8%	•	Vitamin C 4%
Calcium 20%	•	Iron 20%

* Percent Daily Values are based on a 2000 calorie diet. Your daily values may be higher or lower depending on your calorie needs.

One McDonald's cheeseburger.

Serving Size is *1 burger*. Makes sense. They even display the number of grams in that size, 114 grams. *Total Carbohydrate* is 33 grams of which *Sugars* are 7 grams. Now, there are a few grams of *Trans Fat*, 0.4 grams. Not too bad. Let's apply the formula of total grams of carbohydrates *as a percentage* of total grams of food in a serving size: 33 / 114 = 29%. A single McDonald's cheeseburger is composed of about 29% of carbohydrates and contains very few trans-fats. Pretty cool, huh? You can play all kinds of games with the Nutritional Facts of most foods. You can gain a lot of useful LCHF information.

Fast-food chains provide Nutritional Facts for *all* of their foods, often on a single sheet. Finding the Nutritional Facts sheets is pretty easy and they are usually available as a PDF file. Just do a

Google search of "nutritional facts [name of fast-food]."

If you want to permanently save the file, just go to your web browser and select File/Save As. Then, save the file to your Desktop (or wherever) remembering to first change the file name to something appropriate (e.g. McDonald's NF).

Plan your meal *before* you go to a fast-food restaurant. Choose foods with the fewest carbohydrates. Or, bring your iPad along and look up the foods right there. Of course, this'll piss off the people in line behind you.

Portion Sizes

This one's important. Almost everything I've read states that larger portion sizes are the reason Americans are getting fatter.

I disagree. Larger portions are not the *reason* we're getting fatter. Larger portions are a *symptom* of eating too many carbohydrates.

Say what? First, let's explore a possible origin of larger sizes or portions. There's a business-legend that's been floating around for years. Supposedly back in the 1950s, some bright guy approached a toothpaste manufacturer and told them that for $100,000 he could increase toothpaste sales by 40% with almost no increase in production costs. The company executives were skeptical and said they'd get back to him. For two weeks the executives, engineers and scientists of the company conferred, but to no avail. They couldn't come up with an idea that would produce these results. They called the bright guy back, hired and paid him. After a moment, the bright guy handed a small envelope to the CEO. The CEO opened the envelope, took out the small note within and read the words, "Make the hole bigger."

A regular-sized soft drink in the 1950s was 7 ounces. Today you can buy a Double-Gulp containing 64 ounces. I believe that portion sizes were *first* increased as a method to increase sales. I believe that portion sizes were *later* increased due to consumer demand. The increase in serving size was in response to a sort of *energy-demand-loop*. It's kind of like becoming addicted to heroin. You get that great initial *high,* then chase that high for the rest of your life.

The bodies of consumers *liked* these new larger sizes. More energy was available to be consumed. However, because these foods contained larger quantities of carbohydrates, these larger sizes caused more energy to be *stored*. Because this new energy was stored, energy needs weren't met. Consumers now needed even larger sizes. Fast-food companies responded to consumer demands, introducing even larger sizes. Consumers now consumed even more energy. More of the new energy was stored. Consumer demand rose even further. To meet consumer demand, fast-food companies began to produce sizes like *King-Size, Super-Size, Big Gulp* and *Double Gulp*. More and more energy was stored. Folks got fatter and fatter.

This cycle is an *energy-demand-loop* resulting from increasing consumer demand. Fast-food companies aren't evil. They're entities in business to make a profit and make that profit by meeting consumer demand. If fast-food companies were only creating larger serving sizes to increase sales and margin, why haven't we seen *Bucket-Size* or even *55-Gallon-Drum-Size* soft drinks? Hey, KFC does sell a *Bucket* of chicken, but hopefully that size won't be consumed by a single person.

If LCHF gains traction, maybe the food industry will respond to customer demand by reducing serving sizes. With LCHF, folks won't be as hungry or thirsty as they used to be.

Snacking

The reason snacking has increased is the same reason portion sizes have increased. We're eating foods that contain too many carbohydrates causing us to store energy. Our energy needs aren't met. Our bodies tell us to consume more food, *even between meals*. We're stuck in that damn *energy-demand-loop* again.

Supplements and Medication

I take very few supplements and no medication.

In the morning, I take a multivitamin designed for people over the age of 50. I also take 400 I.U. of Vitamin E and 2,000 mg of fish oil with Omega-3. At night I take a second dose of 2,000 mg of fish oil with Omega-3. These supplements seem to benefit my health. They may or may not do the same for you. If you're considering adding a supplement to your diet, do the research.

Congress passed the *Dietary Supplement Act* in 1992. The act prevents the FDA from using its labeling rules on dietary supplements. I'm not sure why anyone would desire a bill *preventing* you from obtaining information about what you're going to put into your body.

With LCHF you won't need to take near as much medication. You should be able to cut back after obtaining your doctor's blessing.

Let's Move!

First Lady Michelle Obama, the incumbent President's spouse, championed a campaign to end childhood obesity called *Let's Move!*

The program promotes "healthy" eating, exercise, consumer power and interaction with pediatricians. *Let's Move!* stresses activity, eating in moderation and eating a *mix* of foods as in those foods found in *MyPlate*[26].

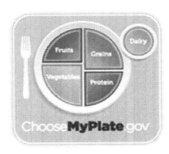

MyPlate was released by the USDA in 2011, replacing *MyPyramid* of 2005, which replaced the *Food Guide Pyramid* of 1992.

---

26 www.choosemyplate.gov

Look at the *Grains* section of the pie. Why is this even included? Hasn't anyone in the current administration even explored the possibility of low-carbohydrate eating?

With LCHF you don't *force* your body to eat in moderation as *MyPlate* suggests. With LCHF you'll begin to eat in moderation with *no effort*. Your systems and cells will function as they've been designed to function.

Let's look at what *Let's Move!* is asking us to feed our children. Here's a Sample Menu taken from *MyPlate Sample Menus*[27]. Go to the link below to see a PDF file of the actual menus being promoted.

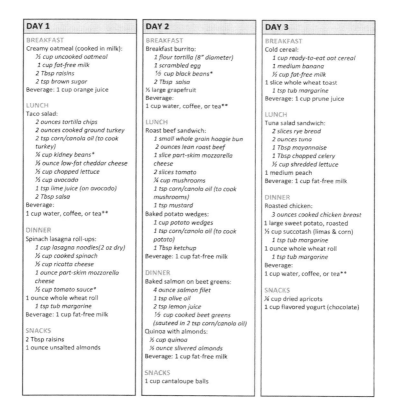

---

27 www.choosemyplate.gov/food-groups/downloads/Sample_Menus-2000Cals-DG2010.pdf

Look at all the carbohydrates they're suggesting we feed our children.

My Plate Sample Menus

· **Breakfast:** Oatmeal, raisins, brown sugar, orange juice, tortillas and toast

· **Lunch:** Chips, buns, potatoes and rye bread

· **Dinner:** Noodles, rolls and sweet potatoes

· **Snacks:** Raisins, cantaloupe, apricots and even yogurt.

Man, did they get it wrong. It's not even close. The kids on this diet will *stay* obese. Oh, they might initially lose weight, but if they ingest carbohydrates, they'll eventually put it back on. All those carbohydrates those obese children are eating will have their fat cells *storing* energy rather than *using* energy.

Maybe, just maybe, LCHF will gain real traction and *Let's Move!* can be modified to incorporate LCHF. That demon obesity will never again harm another child.

As much as the *Tea Party* hates the policies of the Obama Administration, maybe we could get them to protest *Let's Move!* The protest could be centered on replacing the carbohydrates in *Let's Move!* with saturated fats. I know those *Tea Party* guys gotta be meat eaters.

ODDS AND ENDS

"Random thoughts."

Dreaming

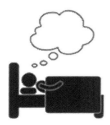

I don't know if it's LCHF, but since eating this way, I dream a lot more. My dreams are vivid. The dreams are in full color and contain plot and subplot. Some of the dreams are so realistic, I have no trouble remembering them.

Energy Ripple

Since I've gone on LCHF, I often experience ripples of energy. Whenever I hear a good piece of music or a great line in a movie, whenever something moves me, ripples of energy run down my spine and the back of my legs. I get these mini-orgasms several times a day. They're wonderful.

Inspirational Times

It always surprises me how many times I'd get a great idea for this book while I showered. I'd often have to finish up quickly, towel off and rush to my iMac to get the thought down. I almost bought a grease pencil to write on the ceramic tile walls. Other times of inspiration were when I'd drank too much red wine with my meal. When on this red-wine-buzz, I'd furiously take notes then try to read them the next day. The notes were often indecipherable.

Contrast Eating

One thing I learned early in life is that food tastes better when eaten in contrasts. Eat something sweet with something salty. Eat something sweet with something bitter. Use *contrast eating* with LCHF. Eat salty bacon followed by a piece of sweet fruit. I used *contrast eating* on Thanksgiving when I ate that sweet pie followed by that bitter coffee.

How to Eat a Big Mac While on LCHF

Once in a great while, I crave a McDonald's Big Mac. I do *adjust* the sandwich before eating. I try to reduce the number of carbohydrates in the sandwich. Step 1: Throw away the top bun. Step 2: Reverse the middle bun and beef patty so that it now becomes the top bun. You end up with a sandwich with very thin top and bottom buns and two hamburger patties in the middle. My guess is the number of carbohydrates is reduced by 40%.

My Friend's Cooking

I've got a friend who lives in the California Delta. She's an amazing person and an autodidact gourmet. Whenever you're invited to her home for a meal, you always accept, even if you already have other plans. This old gal can cook, really cook. One time she introduced me to grilled portabella mushrooms. One bite and I thought I was eating steak. My guess is that there are many alternatives to eating meat for those vegetarians choosing LCHF.

LCHF Antipasto Dinner

One of the things I occasionally like to have for dinner is a meal of *antipasto*, an appetizer typically consisting of olives, cured meats and cheeses. I treat this Italian appetizer as a meal. I prepare a plate of salami, pastrami, prosciutto, various cheeses, a little fruit, pickles and most importantly, olives. This "dinner" is very LCHF friendly and tastes great, especially when consumed with a few glasses of soft, red wine. My friend, Julia and I would often share this meal.

Snacks

In Thailand I often shop at Makro, a warehouse club comparable to Costco in its infancy. I recently decided to review the carbohydrates contained in snacks. There are several aisles containing various snacks. I focused on the huge aisle containing *Extruded Corn Snacks*. The nutritional labeling was entirely in Thai except for the word "carbohydrates." Each small bag of *Extruded Corn Snacks* contained 18 grams of carbohydrates. What really surprised me were the ingredients. The snacks were composed almost entirely of corn *starch*. Not corn *flour*, but corn *starch*. I just wish they didn't taste so damn good.

7-Eleven Mashed Potato Vending Machine

It seems that in some countries, 7-Eleven is selling mashed potatoes and gravy by way of a vending machine. Do a Google search if you don't believe me. That's what we need, more carbohydrates from 7-Eleven.

Low Self-esteem

Low self-esteem is often listed as a reason for overeating. Folks that don't think much of themselves are thought to overeat as a way to counteract their feelings of limited self-worth. If you have low self-esteem, carbohydrates may be a contributing factor. Give them up and switch to saturated fats. You won't feel like overeating any more. Your self-esteem may rise.

Obese Babies

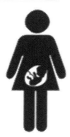

I recently found out that many babies are now obese. Huh? How the hell can that be? It seems that if a woman consumes carbohydrates during her pregnancy, the harmful effects of those carbohydrates are passed on to the fetus. The babies are born with cells that don't function as they should. The carbohydrates have caused the babies to produce insulin even while they're in the womb. This one really blew me away. It also made a lot of sense. We strongly discourage pregnant mothers from smoking cigarettes or drinking alcohol as both are passed on to the fetus. Why not discourage pregnant mothers from eating carbohydrates?

Herpes

I have a friend who suffers from genital herpes. He had a small outbreak of the virus about twice a year. Since going on LCHF, he hasn't had a single outbreak.

Adjustable Gastric Band

Being morbidly obese must be a terrible psychological burden. If you're willing to subject yourself to the insertion of a *Gastric Band*, you're pretty screwed up.

Years ago I was visiting my mother, sister and niece at their home in California. My niece had brought a friend home, a very pretty 20 year-old woman who was morbidly obese. The friend told us that she was about to undergo surgery and have a *Gastric Band* put in place. She explained that due to her young age, she had to strongly lobby her doctor to get him to agree to the procedure. It's too bad I didn't know about LCHF back then.

Menstrual Complications

It didn't take much research to confirm this, but it seems that eating LCHF alters a woman's menstrual cycle. Eating LCHF will result in menstrual cycles that are lighter and shorter. A woman eating LCHF will have less bloating and cramping. This is reason enough to get onboard.

Peeing in the Dark

My family must be missing some key food-processing enzyme. We're a gassy bunch. When we'd all get together, the eruption of gas following a big meal was kind of daunting. As I got older, this gas production became a problem. At night it would trick my body into thinking I had to pee. Several times a night, the pressure of the gas against my bladder would cause me to awaken. I'd sleepily advance to the toilet, squirt out a tiny bit of urine, expel gas, return to bed and hopefully to sleep. Since going on LCHF, this rarely happens. Why? My guess is that it's because my visceral fat has shrunk. There's more room for the gas. I think I've just found the reason I sleep better on LCHF, fewer nightly wake ups.

Roger Maris

I recently watched the movie 61* for the third or fourth time. The movie deals with the 1961 race between Mickey Mantel and Roger Maris in trying to break Babe Ruth's home run record of 60. In the movie, Roger Maris eats some terrible looking green bacon and eggs. He claims that this meal improves his time at bat. Roger persuades Mickey to try the same meal. Mickey's time at bat improves. Supposedly, this scene is based upon fact. I found this quote in an article by Harvey Frommer.

> *"When Roger Maris was going for the home run record he would eat only bologna and eggs for breakfast," Roger's friend Julie Isaacson recalled. "Every morning we would have breakfast together at the Stage Deli."*

Mickey and Roger didn't know it, but they were using LCHF to chase the Babe's record.

Watching Movies in the U.S.

About once a year, I try to visit my sister and niece at their home in California. Both my sister and I enjoy going to the movies. Whenever I visit, we often go together. I hadn't gone to the movies in the U.S. for some time, so when I ordered popcorn and a soft drink, I was surprised at the serving sizes. A *regular size* was enormous, much more than I could consume. I ended up buying the *children's size*.

Watching Movies Abroad

This one has nothing to do with LCHF. It's just an observation of living abroad. I enjoy watching movies at home and I enjoy sharing the experience with others. This is true for my time in both Costa Rica and Thailand. There are many movies available in both countries that contain subtitles, Spanish for Costa Rica and Thai for Thailand. Many of the movies also offer a local-language *audio* track. It's a little odd hearing Tom Cruise and Jack Nicholson yelling at one another in Thai (try Google Translate).

> *Kaffee:* ฉันต้องการความจริง
>
> *Jessup:* คุณไม่สามารถจัดการความจริง
>
> *- Lt. Kaffee to Col. Jessup in A Few Good Men (1992), as played by Tom Cruise and Jack Nicholson*

I'd try to choose a movie that I thought might appeal to the woman I was with. Romantic comedies or light slapstick. These movies were usually met with approval, but not as much as I'd expected. The movies that go over big are the movies that went over big from decades past. *Quality is timeless and without borders.* Surprisingly, *The Wizard of Oz (1939)* is always well received as are *Jaws (1975)*, *The Shawshank Redemption (1994)* and *Cinderella Man (2005)*.

Without exception, the #1 favorite in both Costa Rica and Thailand is *Pretty Woman (1990)*. Most of the women I entertain are from poor backgrounds. They often have limited resources and education. Is it any wonder they hope to become Vivian Ward (Julia Roberts) and find their own Edward Lewis (Richard Gere)? They also all love *Sex and the City (1998-2004)*, probably for the same reason. Do you know how many times I've been called *"Meesta Beeg"*?

FINISHING TOUCHES

"Challenge, evaluate, accept."

Recap

Your body needs energy to function. That need can be satisfied with carbohydrates or saturated fats.

Saturated fats are good for you. Your body is designed to process them. Saturated fats help your body to *use* energy. Saturated fats improve your cognitive ability and your blood chemistry. Saturated fats help men produce testosterone and women produce estrogen. Saturated fats improve your life.

Carbohydrates are bad for you. Your body is *not* designed to process them. Carbohydrates cause your body to *store* energy. Carbohydrates cause inflammation and insulin production. Carbohydrates cause you to become lethargic and harm your blood chemistry. Carbohydrates harm your life.

Using LCHF, you replace carbohydrates with saturated fats. You'll lose weight and your health will improve. You'll have more energy and your sex life will improve. You'll gain many benefits and you'll never have to exercise or feel starved.

It seems to be an easy choice.

Leading Causes of Death in the U.S.

The data from 2009, the last year calculated, shows the following as the *Leading Causes of Death* in the United States.

Leading Causes of Death

- Heart disease: 599,413

- Cancer: 567,628

- Chronic lower respiratory diseases: 137,353

- Stroke (cerebrovascular diseases): 128,842

- Accidents (unintentional injuries): 118,021

- Alzheimer's disease: 79,003

- Diabetes: 68,705

- Influenza and Pneumonia: 53,692

- Nephritis, nephrotic syndrome, and nephrosis: 48,935
- Intentional self-harm (suicide): 36,909

Hopefully you've gained a lot of knowledge about the harm carbohydrates can cause.

Go down this list and apply the knowledge you've gained.

Skepticism

I am an admitted fanatic when it comes to eating LCHF. I try to get everyone I know eating LCHF. Many of my friends have embraced this way of eating. However, there are always skeptics. Many times my discussions are met with folded arms and looks of disdain. Some guys are just not willing to change or even listen.

One friend, a 62 year-old retired U.S. Marine officer, showed no interest whatsoever in LCHF. He would *pooh-pooh* pretty much anything I said concerning LCHF. When I told him that LCHF gave me an HDL cholesterol level of 102, he simply didn't believe me. I had to show him the actual blood test results.

My friend has always been one of those powerful, stocky men, usually about 25 pounds overweight. I recently ran into my friend. I hadn't seen him in a month or so. The guy looked great. It was obvious he'd lost weight. When I asked him how he did it, his response was, "I tried your damn diet." Then he grinned and bought me a drink.

I have another friend here, "Big Dick Steve," a 50 year-old retired software executive from New York. This guy is fun to be with. He's big, loud and very funny. He's also the biggest skeptic I know. This guy has been overweight for a very long time. He's one of those former athletes. Still very powerful and muscled, but now wearing thick layers of subcutaneous fat. He's a big guy, about 300 pounds. He could lose about 80 of those pounds.

"Big Dick Steve" has a very strong *Type-A* personality. He won't take advice from anyone unless he thinks the advice was his to begin with. He knows how successful LCHF has been with me and other members of our circle. He knows, but he still wants to go *old school*. He recently telephoned me and told me of his plans to workout and limit his caloric intake to about 1,000-1,500 per day. I think he thought I'd be impressed.

This guy normally eats more than anyone I know. It's not uncommon for him to order three breakfasts at the same time. Of course he washes everything down with a soft drink, "Ey' ya, gimme CoCola." He's somehow turned Coca Cola into a single word.

You and I both know what's going to happen. He's going to lose a lot of weight, then put it back on in 2 or 3 months. His fat cells are used to extended *periods of gluttony*. Now he's going to put those fat cells into a *period of famine*. The fat cells will grudgingly give up their stored energy through his starvation and exercise, but the next time he eats a big meal, those same fat cells will lock down hard.

I really like Steve. It's a joy to be around him and his infectious laughter. I truly hope the best for him, but my guess is that he's a lost cause.

The single funniest thing I've ever seen Steve do is when he gave a *wai*, the traditional Thai greeting, to a baby elephant. Steve and I were carousing in the little town of Baan Chang here in Thailand. As we were about to enter a bar, we noticed a Thai man leading a baby elephant down the street. You could buy bananas or sugar cane from the man and feed them to his elephant. Steve had never been that close to an elephant, so he bought all the treats. The elephant ate them all.

When Steve was finished feeding the elephant, he gave the baby elephant a *wai*. He pressed his palms together, faced the elephant and bowed. The damn elephant bowed its head and returned the *wai*.

Steve gave the elephant a second *wai*. The elephant again responded. My friend gave another and another, rapidly increasing the number of *wais*. The elephant answered each and every *wai*.

Here were these two giant creatures, my hysterically laughing 300 pound friend and the baby 2,000 pound elephant, rapidly bowing their heads at one another. All the bars cleared out to watch. It was damned funny.

Of course bananas and sugar cane both contain carbohydrates. Maybe that's why elephants are so big.

I have one final skeptic to discuss. Every Sunday morning I eat an LCHF breakfast at *Rich Man Poor Man*, an expat restaurant and hotel. The place is owned by a 50 year-old Yankee fan named Eddie. I like Eddie. I consider him to be a good friend. He's loud, funny and about 40 pounds overweight. Eddie is kind enough to alter his meals to accommodate his customers on LCHF. He willingly exchanges the toast and potatoes for an extra egg. Eddie knows there are 4 or 5 of us eating LCHF. He's seen the results. He's seen us all getting slimmer and healthier. I think he hates the results. Every time anyone brings up LCHF, he ridicules it. He tells us that there is no way we can keep this up. He tells us that we'll eventually go back to eating carbohydrates. He tells us that what we're eating is unhealthy. I always respond with something like, "Hey Eddie, it's OK. Even though I've been on LCHF for 18 months and I get better every day, you don't have to try it. Some guys don't mind being fat."

I'm always surprised at how defensive some folks are. They either doubt the veracity of what I tell them about LCHF, or they think it's just another *fad-diet* that will help them quickly lose weight then put it right back on.

It often takes me more than a few conversations until the logic of LCHF begins to overcome their preconceived notions. When they finally get onboard, the results are always better than they'd ever imagined.

The Prospect

A good friend of mine, *Wild Bill* Wichrowski, is one of the newer captains on *Deadliest Catch*[28], a popular Discovery Channel show about crab fishing.

We were in the U.S. Navy together in the late 1970s. Over the last 30 years, we've had a lot of fun and gotten into a lot of trouble

---

28 dsc.discovery.com/tv/deadliest-catch/

together. He's a hard-drinking, hard-fighting kind of guy. He's very smart and very funny. Women love him.

We've stayed friends over the years. In the late 1990s, he would come down from Alaska and visit me at my home in the California Delta, a series of rivers and sloughs perfect for waterskiing and jet skiing.

He would always bring seafood with him on his visits, 50 pounds of king crab, 50 pounds of salmon and 50 pounds of halibut. This guy is a good cook, good enough to host a huge neighborhood feast at my home. When word got out, my telephone would be ringing away with neighbors requesting invites.

Each neighbor or two would be required to bring a bottle of chilled Jaegermeister as an *entrance fee* to the shindig. I'd use Smurf Dixie Cups as shot glasses, filling dozens of the cups on my counter. Most of my neighbors were in their 50s and 60s, all retired, but these guys and gals could party.

My friend would prepare some amazing dishes. Herbed salmon steamed over orange slices. Baked halibut made with crushed pineapple, brown-sugar, fennel, onions and bacon. Of course he always served crabs legs with melted butter. The feasts were always amazing.

When I first met Bill in 1978, he was very slim, maybe 6'3" 180 pounds. On his visits to the Delta he was somewhat bigger, maybe 220 pounds. A few years later, he would visit me in Costa Rica, this time even bigger, about 240 pounds. I watched a recent episode of *Deadliest Catch* and he's really big. Maybe 260 pounds. This friend is my next *prospect*. I like him and his company very much. I hope to get him on LCHF and get him back to fighting weight.

Offer of Withdrawal

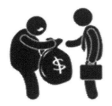

If this book ever gains traction, I expect attacks from the food and pharmaceutical giants. I want these giants to know that I *can* be bought. Cut me the right deal and I'll yank this puppy from the electronic bookshelves faster than you can down a Fun-Size bag of M&Ms. The deal better be pretty sweet [smile].

Eighteen Months of LCHF

As of the time of this writing, I've been on LCHF for 18 months. During that time, my body has changed a lot. I'm not a vain person, I rarely look in the mirror, yet, I find myself doing so lately. As most men age, their stomach *increases* in size and protrudes. As most men age, their buttocks *decrease* in size, becoming smaller and flatter. We eventually end up wearing our wallets on the "back of our knee." LCHF has reversed this trend for me. My stomach is smaller and oddly, my buttocks are larger. I've lost the visceral fat that made my stomach protrude. I've also lost much of the subcutaneous fat in my buttocks, yet my *glutes* have firmed up and gotten larger. I now look in the mirror and ask myself, "Who the hell is that guy? He looks pretty good." When I first got on LCHF, I noticed major changes in weight loss, energy and health. I very quickly got slimmer, felt better and had more energy. Then I hit a downward sloping plateau. I still got slimmer and healthier, but at a much slower pace. That is, until recently. Almost overnight, my body really improved. My body is now much the same as it was when I was 20 years old. I was 187 pounds then and I'm 187 pounds now. I did this all without ever starving or exercise. I did this all with LCHF.

Closing Statement

I've tried to present you with a book that's interesting, informative and accurate. Much of what you've read is based upon the results of clinical studies. Much of what you've read is my conjecture, supposition and association. Whenever I made a guess, an estimate or projected a hypothesis, I tried to let you know.

Challenge what I've written. Challenge "medical authorities," your doctor included. Many "medical authorities" are unaware of recent clinical findings and cling to that old-school mantra, "Fats are bad for you." Challenge these dinosaurs. Do your own research. Try to find arguments both for and against LCHF. Make an informed decision about what you put into your body.

I do believe that LCHF can help anyone. LCHF has improved my life in many ways. LCHF has improved the lives of many of my friends. LCHF can improve your life.

If you embrace LCHF, don't be surprised if you begin viewing life through *LCHF Goggles*. You'll know the carbohydrate content of every food you see. You'll assess what your friends are eating. You'll assess what television characters are eating. You'll even assess what types of body fat folks are carrying around.

You'll drive all of your friends and family crazy.

It's kinda fun.

If you've embraced LCHF, spread the word. Get those you love on LCHF. Hell, get them to buy this book directly from my site, **loseweightwithlchf.com**. God I'm shameless.

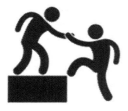

APPENDIX

There are three sources that had the most influence on what I put into this book:

(1) The documentary, "Fat Head," by Tom Naughton.

(2) An LCHF video lecture by Dr. Andreas Eenfeldt.

(3) A series of video lectures by Dr. Robert Lustig.

Fat Head

I've watched *Fat Head*, the rebuttal to *Super Size Me*, several times. I gain additional information with each viewing. I strongly suggest you take a look at *Fat Head*.

I'd only watched *Super Size Me* one time, right after the movie was first produced. The movie made an impact on me and was strongly received by the public. However, *Fat Head* made such a great rebuttal to *Super Size Me*, that I didn't wish to bother with it a second time.

This was a mistake. I recently decided to watch *Super Size Me* a second time, but now armed with better knowledge about carbohydrates and fats.

In *Super Size Me,* Morgan Spurlock gains a lot of weight and his health dramatically declines. He blames McDonald's food. I now know that it wasn't that he was eating at McDonald's three times a day that produced these harmful results, it was that he had *tripled* the number of carbohydrates he consumed every day that produced these harmful results.

All the bad health trends Morgan discusses in the movie, obesity, childhood diabetes, ADD and many others, are the result of the increase of carbohydrates in the American diet, a diet that's now worldwide.

Finish reading this book and then try to watch both *Fat Head* and *Super Size Me* again. This time try focusing on what you've learned about the effects of carbohydrates.

The oddest thing about watching *Super Size Me* is that I really craved a Big Mac both times I watched it.

Tom Naughton has a website worth checking out, *Fat Head*[29]. The site doesn't deal with the movie very much as the site-address implies but Tom provides a lot of current information concerning low-carbohydrate eating. Besides his site, Tom has also given several lectures, most available on YouTube.

When I first began my research on LCHF, I contacted Mr. Naughton and was happily surprised when he responded to my emails. Tom has helped me better understand many of the aspects of low-carbohydrate eating.

The Diet Doctor

The LCHF movement is really gaining ground in Sweden and other Scandinavian countries. There were many debates in Sweden, both public and private, concerning LCHF. The results of these debates were so positive that much of the population has embraced the LCHF style of eating. Public health in Sweden is steadily improving.

One of the advocates there is a doctor by the name of Dr. Andreas Eenfeldt. I first became aware of Dr. Eenfeldt after watching a video of him giving a lecture at the Ancestral Health Symposium.

This video is very comprehensive, informative and entertaining. It can be found on YouTube by doing a search of "The Food Revolution" or on Dr. Eenfeldt's website, *The Diet Doctor*[30]. The site is nicely laid out and available in English, Swedish, Danish, German and Hebrew. I suggest you try the doctor's introductory *LCHF for Beginners*[31] first.

Surprisingly, Dr. Eenfeldt has responded to my emails. He's provided me with answers to several questions concerning LCHF. He's been polite and happy to share. Try his site to gain a lot of pertinent information on LCHF.

---

29 www.fathead-movie.com
30 www.dietdoctor.com
31 www.dietdoctor.com/lchf

The Skinny on Obesity

Do a search on YouTube for "The Skinny on Obesity" or go directly to the site *UCTV Prime*[32] and view it there. Dr. Robert Lustig, a Pediatric Endocrinologist from the University of California, San Francisco, presents this amazing set of seven lectures. These lectures emphasize the science behind limiting the intake of carbohydrates. I've watched these lectures many times. I gain something new with each viewing.

Low-Carb Websites to Explore

The low-carbohydrate movement grows every day. Websites are beginning to reflect this growth. As I wrote this book, I used various medical studies, medical articles, low-carbohydrate websites and blogs as sources. I offer my apologies as I didn't properly catalog my sources. Below you'll find links to many of these websites and blogs. I've listed them in alphabetical order. Explore these websites, obtain differing views. Find the common link; the dangers of eating carbohydrates.

Dr. Anika Dahlqvist - **annikadahlqvistblogenglish.blogspot.com**

Archevore - **www.archevore.com**

The Atkins Foundation - **www.atkinsfoundation.org**

Blood Sugar 101 - **www.phlaunt.com/diabetes/**

Carb Wars Cookbook - **carbwars.blogspot.com**

Carbohydrates Can Kill - **www.carbohydratescankill.com**

Cholesterol and Health - **www.cholesterol-and-health.com**

Chris Kresser - **chriskresser.com/beyondpaleo**

Connect Nutrition - **www.connectnutrition.com**

Controlled Carbohydrate Nutrition - **www.controlcarb.com**

Cooking Caveman - **cookingcaveman.tumblr.com**

D-solve - **www.dsolve.com**

Diabetes Health - **www.diabeteshealth.com**

Diet Doctor - **www.dietdoctor.com**

---

32 www.uctv.tv/skinny-on-obesity/

Dr. Biffa - **www.drbriffa.com**

The Eating Academy - **eatingacademy.com**

Fat Head - **www.fathead-movie.com**

Fit to the Finish - **www.fittothefinish.com/blog/**

Food Politics - **www.foodpolitics.com**

Fooducate - **www.fooducate.com**

Freckle's Food - **frecklesfood.blogspot.com**

Free the Animal - **freetheanimal.com**

Gary Taubes - **garytaubes.com**

HALO Research - **www.haloresearch.ca**

Healthy Eating Politics - **www.healthy-eating-politics.com**

Hold the Toast - **holdthetoast.com**

Hunt Gather Love - **huntgatherlove.com**

Hunter-Gatherer - **hunter-gatherer.com**

Hyperlipid - **high-fat-nutrition.blogspot.com**

It's Not About Nutrition - **itsnotaboutnutrition.squarespace.com**

LCHF.com - **www.lchf.com**

Left Coast LCHF - **leftcoastlchf.net**

Livin' La Vida LowCarb - **livinlavidalowcarb.com/blog/**

Living an Optimized Life - **jackkruse.com**

Low Carb Diets - **lowcarbdiets.about.com**

Low Carb Friends - **www.lowcarbfriends.com**

Low Carb High Fat USA - **lowcarbhighfatusa.blogspot.com**

Low Carb Luxury - **www.lowcarbluxury.com**

Mark's Daily Apple - **www.marksdailyapple.com**

Matt Metzgar - **www.mattmetzgar.com**

Nutrition and Metabolism Society - **www.nmsociety.org**

Obesity Panacea - **blogs.plos.org/obesitypanacea/**

The Paleo Diet - **thepaleodiet.com**

Protein Power - **www.proteinpower.com**

Second Opinions - **www.second-opinions.co.uk**

Self Nutrition Data - **nutritiondata.self.com**

Serious Strength - **www.seriousstrength.com/site/**

The Skinny on Obesity - **www.uctv.tv/skinny-on-obesity/**

Summer Tomato - **summertomato.com**

Tummyrumble - **www.tummyrumble.net**

U.S. Food Policy - **usfoodpolicy.blogspot.com**

University of South Florida - **www.usf.edu**

The Weston A. Price Foundation - **www.westonaprice.org**

Whole Health Source - **wholehealthsource.blogspot.com**

Writing Conventions I Used

There are many ways to use "quotation marks," *italics* and abbreviations. I chose ways I find most visually pleasing and tried to remain consistent throughout this work.

LCHF = Low-Carb-High-Fat

Low-Carbohydrate-High-Fat can be stated in four different ways:

- · LCHF
- · L.C.H.F.
- · Low-Carb-High-Fat
- · Low-Carbohydrate-High-Fat.

The four are synonymous. I used LCHF as it was easiest to type and is easiest to read.

"Quotation marks" and Italics

I've used "quotation marks" in the following situations:

- · When dialogue is indicated
- · When nicknames are used
- · When sarcasm is implied (e.g. "healthy" snacks)
- · When illustrating a Google, YouTube or Wikipedia search
- · When quotes are given

I've used *italics* in the following situations:

· When emphasis is desired
· When jargon is used
· When slang is used
· When non-English words are used
· When uncommon scientific terms are given
· When uncommon medical terms are given
· When the title of a work is given
· When photo captions are included
· When quotes are given

Privacy

In many of the anecdotes I refer to a subject as *my friend* or *my relative*. I did this rather than using the subject's name for reasons of privacy. If you see an individual's name, it's because I was given the OK to use it.

Quotes

Quotes with no names beneath them are my own or are unattributed.

Book Cover Design

It took me several long, taxing days to design the logos, book covers, front and back, and write the text within. One of the things I pondered over was which logo to use on the front cover. I sent out 3 drafts to various friends and asked them which logo they preferred. The votes were all over the place, almost equally divided. The 3 choices can be seen on the following page.

A Thai friend of mine was visiting me as I designed the book cover. I asked her which logo she preferred and what she thought each logo meant. She immediately chose Logo #1, the overweight man looking down at the scale. She said Logo #1 meant, "Not get fat." She said Logo #2, the man eating a burger and fries, meant, "Not eat." She wasn't sure about Logo #3, the standing overweight man, and said, "*Mai lu.*," Thai for "I don't know."

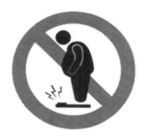

Logo #1

Logo #2

Logo #3

I eventually settled on Logo #1. Which logo would you have picked?

Contacting Me

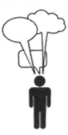

I welcome any thoughts or comments, both positive *and* negative. I can be reached at **eric@loseweightwithlchf.com**.

Tell me what you think, good or bad. Don't hold back, I can take it. I especially welcome specific tales of how LCHF has changed your life. Your stories might end up in the sequel.

32057148R00093

Made in the USA
Lexington, KY
05 May 2014